baby mama
DRAMA

Law and Medicine

Chandra Jones MD, FACOG

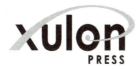

Copyright © 2015 by Chandra Jones MD, FACOG

Baby Mamma Drama
Law and Medicine
by Chandra Jones MD, FACOG

Printed in the United States of America

ISBN 9781498439152

All rights reserved solely by the author. The author guarantees all contents are original and do not infringe upon the legal rights of any other person or work. No part of this book may be reproduced in any form without the permission of the author. The views expressed in this book are not necessarily those of the publisher.

Scripture quotations taken from the New Living Translation (NLT). Copyright © 2004 by Tyndale House Foundation. Used by permission. All rights reserved.

www.xulonpress.com

Foreword

In *Baby Mama Drama: Law and Medicine,* Dr. Jones presents a captivating, entertaining and educational story in an effective and compelling manner. Dr. Jones addresses issues associated with life, death and morbidity. She writes on health topics that relate both to the patients who are depicted in her novel and the health challenges that the central character encounters. The novel opens with this main character, Dr. Jones, being treated by her own physician. By relating to her own health issues, she positions her readers to identify better with the story line. As an obstetrician, Dr. Jones is responsible for obstetric patients and holds additional responsibility for these patients' unborn children.

The author is well prepared professionally for this responsibility. She is trained and board certified in the medical discipline of obstetrics and gynecology, and she has completed sub-specialty training in maternal and fetal medicine (high-risk obstetrics). She most recently conducted her practice through the obstetrics and gynecology service of the Kings County Hospital in Brooklyn, New York. Without question, the training and skills Dr. Jones possesses are essential for her to successfully address the myriad of medical challenges that emerge in this high-risk service. Thus, she is ideally suited to write this novel.

The novel describes the numerous extremely challenging health scenarios that tax Dr. Jones both medically and emotionally. As such, the title *Baby Mama Drama* is most fitting. Additionally, she has to relate to the family members of her patients. Her responses to patients and their families range from that of absolute firmness to outright humor. Dr. Jones realizes that different responses are dictated by the varying nature of the personalities and temperaments of the individuals she encounters. This understanding of human nature is necessary, not only in her interactions with patients and their family members, but also within her interactions with her co-workers. Her relationships with co-workers, which are not always amicable, are chronicled in several of the storylines. It is not unusual for some of the patients that Dr. Jones encounters to have their own agendas, especially when pain control medications are involved. But Dr. Jones is almost always shrewd enough to avoid being hoodwinked. Furthermore, throughout the book she demonstrates the capacity to adapt to situations appropriately and does so quite adroitly. Thus, the author clearly demonstrates her understanding of both the science and the art of medicine. In addressing the numerous medical emergencies described in the book, she uses diagrams and anatomical drawings that are clear and unambiguous. This brings clarity to the topics discussed. Indeed, the extent of the information she offers provides an education to readers who are not trained in medicine.

Dr. Jones gives this book energy by assigning each character a distinctive personality, which creates excitement as she interacts with them. The scenes in the book move briskly, are focused and leave the reader impatiently awaiting the next episode—truly what a good book does. I recommend this book without reservation to those readers who are seeking a spirited and entertaining book to read. Finally, I am grateful to Dr. Jones for writing this book and am most appreciative of the enjoyment it has brought me.

Henry W. Foster, Jr., MD, FACOG
Professor *Emeritus* & former Dean & Vice
President for Medical Services Meharry
Medical College &
Clinical Professor, Obstetrics & Gynecology Vanderbilt University & Former
Clinton nominee, US Surgeon General

Acknowledgments

For me, the most difficult aspect of producing this inspirational book is writing the acknowledgments

There are so many wonderful people who have come into my life and played a role in making this concept a success. I have been inspired, motivated, encouraged, and given loving criticism, and I count all the input as blessings.

To begin this section most appropriately, I must give credit for the vision, direction and overwhelming success of this project to my God and Father.

It goes without saying that I am thankful to my family, my loving mother, brother, and cousin: Elouise Jones, Michael Jones, and Deborah Davis. I am thankful to my Godparents: Dr. Billy and Dr. Urias Beverly

I am thankful to my extended family: Liska Bodrick, Regenia Harrison-Moore, Hattie Shinault, Romualda Watson, and Steven Marr.

I am thankful to my colleagues and mentors: Yvonne Thornton, MD; Jeanette Thornton, MD; Henry Foster Jr, MD; Wendy Woods, MD, Cheryl Clarke, MD, and B David Blake, MD

I am thankful to my legal family: Judge Mablean Ephriam, Donald Thigpen, Esq, and Robert Higgenbotham.

I am sincerely grateful for the inspiration of this book, which came from Lauren and "Big Boom" Freeman. Their love, support and guidance was greatly appreciated during the really tough times.

A special appreciation is extended to the Xulon Press family and Bookstylings.com for their tireless assistance and devotion to this project.

I would be remiss if I failed to thank Lady Grace Edwards, my church family and Bishop T.D. Jakes of the Potter's House Church in Dallas, Texas, for blessing this project.

There are so many other people who have influenced this work, too many to mention. I hope they know I am grateful for all the support and prayers bestowed upon me during this time of thought and concentration.

Most of all, I thank you, the reader, for making this project a success. I am excited that you chose my work for an avenue of excitement, learning, entertainment, and suspense.

Table of Contents

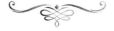

Foreword
    Henry W. Foster, Jr., MD, FACOG v

Acknowledgments vii

Chapters
1. In the Doctor's Office 11
2. Mercy General Hospital 15
3. Breech Delivery 23
4. My Father 43
5. Back to Work 47
6. Mercy General Hospital 51
7. Morning Breakfast 59
8. Memories of Mother 65
9. Driving to the Hospital 69
10. Hospital Entrance 71
11. Mercy General Hospital 75
12. Administration Conference 81
13. Labor and Delivery 85
14. Doctor's Lounge 89
15. Morning Report 93
16. Mother's Accident 95
17. Emergency Services 97
18. Morning Report 101
19. Labor and Delivery 103
20. Emergency Room 105
21. Catastrophe 109

22. Operating Room 113
23. Trauma Surgeons 121
24. No Prenatal Care 125
25. Operating Room 1 129
26. Mrs. Crane Returns 133
27. Neurosurgeons 135
28. Operating Room 137
29. Labor and Delivery 139
30. Emergency Room 143
31. Cliffhanger 145

Appendix

Medical Definitions 149
Medical Specialists 155
Medications 157
Medical Abbreviations 159
Helpful Medical Organizations 161
References 163

Chapter 1

In the Doctor's Office

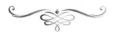

Sitting in the office of my cardiologist always makes me nervous. It is freezing cold in here. I appreciate that the nurse brought me a blanket. I wrap the blanket around the thin little paper drape and look at the walls. I see pictorials of heart disease everywhere. Seeing the cardiologist is like visiting the funeral director: you don't see him unless there is trouble. And that is why I am here... *trouble*.

Dr. Beta enters the room holding my test results in his hand. "Hello, Chandra. How are you doing today?"

"I will know better after you tell me the results of the test."

Dr. Beta asks, "Have you been feeling tired?"

This is a set-up question. This is not starting out good. The look on his face and the concern in his voice acts as a warning; the news is going to be bad.

I think to myself, "I am an obstetrician, overworked, stressed, and always tired."

I say to Dr. Beta, "A little tired sometimes."

"Have you been feeling short of breath or experiencing any chest pain?"

I fight back the tears, and with a squeaky voice reply, "A little; the test results must not be good." I brace myself for the worst.

Dr. Beta holds up the film. "Today's test results show a significant change from last year. Your blood pressure is elevated. Your pressure is trying to compensate for your failing heart. I need to start you on medication right away."

I am in shock. My breathing stops. I feel like a knife has just gone through my chest. I see Dr. Beta's lips moving, but I cannot hear a word he is saying.

"Do you have a blood pressure cuff at home? Chandra, do you have a blood pressure cuff?"

I manage to find the words, "No, Sir."

"Remind me to give you one before you leave. I want you to start monitoring your blood pressure twice a day. Take your pressure in the morning and then again in the afternoon. Keep a blood pressure log and bring it to your next appointment. I want to see you back here in one month. Do you have any questions?"

Do I have any questions? I cannot even think. I am in shock, and my mind has checked out of my body... It has left the building. My poor heart and I are left alone. I look up at Dr. Beta, and with a sound that I don't even recognize, I finally manage to speak, "No Sir, no questions."

Dr. Beta walks up to me and puts his hand on my shoulder. "Could it be that private practice is too stressful for you?" he asks, "I want you to take better care of yourself. It is important that you slow down and keep stress to a minimum."

With nervous hands, I take the prescription. I look up as the tears start to fall. "Thank you, Dr. Beta."

"You are welcome. I will leave the room so you can get dressed."

Hands trembling, I manage to put my clothes back on. I look in the mirror; I look and feel a mess.

I leave the room and walk up to my mother who is sitting in the waiting room. "Mom, I am ready to go."

"Just give me a minute dear. I want to hear the verdict of the judge. This is a good episode."

My mother looks up and sees the pain in my eyes.

"Chandra you don't look so good; we better go. I will have to catch this episode on rerun."

As we leave the waiting room, the lady sitting by the door tells my mother, "The Judge throws the book at that scoundrel."

Mom replies, "I figured as much. He had it coming."

We walk to the car in silence.

"Better let me drive, Chandra."

"Good idea."

I hand my mother the keys and fall into the passenger's seat.

"What did Dr. Beta say?"

"My heart has gotten worst."

"Really? You got that condition from your father. He died of heart problems, his mother died from heart problems, and his father died from heart problems. I don't think anyone on his side of the family lived much past fifty."

"Mom, thanks for the burial update. I know you are just trying to help, but it really is not working. Talking about Dad and all my dead relatives is not my idea of a cheer-up conversation."

"Sorry, I just want you to remember; this heart thing is not your fault. You inherited those bad heart genes from your father. Nobody on my side of the family has any mess like that. We just drop dead from drinking too much liquor and bad diabetes; but, come to think of it, your aunt Pearl did have a baby with a heart problem."

"A heart problem?"

"Yes, the doctor said it was alcohol syndrome. You think that would have scared Pearl straight. But it didn't. Pearl was on that hard liquor. She sobered up just long enough to get through the funeral. After the funeral was over, Pearl went right back to drinking. She drank herself into the ground."

I let out a deep sigh.

"When are you scheduled for surgery?"

The word surgery snaps me back into reality.

"Surgery!"

"Yes, they are doing wonderful things with the human heart these days."

"I know."

"I was watching the Discovery Channel, and I caught a glimpse of some doctors working on a baboon's heart."

"Mom, please no surgery for now. Let's give the medication a chance."

"Did Dr. Beta give you a beta blocker?"

"Yeah."

"That stuff makes you feel like crap. Zaps your energy. Kills your sex drive."

"Mommmm!"

"Is your life insurance and burial policy up to date?"

"Mom, I cannot believe you."

"You know all the confusion we had when we lost your father. It took us two years to pay off the funeral home, and I am still saving my bingo money to get him a stone. The shape he left us in, he deserves a..."

"Mom, let the dead rest in peace."

"Okay, I just want to make sure the same thing does not happen to you in the event you drop dead... I mean, in the event of your early departure."

I cannot believe we are having this conversation. My mother has me in the ground and is trying to collect a check.

"Mom, can we please change the subject?"

"Sorry dear. I will change the subject."

"Mom, can you swing by the pharmacy so I can get my prescription filled?"

"What, the receptionist did not give you any samples? That woman is more interested in gossiping on the phone than doing her job. I have an appointment with Dr. Beta next Friday. Just wait until I tell him. I will get you some samples."

"Mom, they gave me a few samples to get started and a blood pressure monitor. I also have a prescription I need to fill."

"We can drop off your prescription and I can pick it up later. I have some errands to run, and it won't be a problem to pick it up then."

"That sounds like a great idea. I just want to go home and lay down."

"When does Dr. Beta want to see you again?"

"The next appointment is in one month."

"I hope it is on a Friday. Friday is a good day to see the cardiologist. That way, if you have to stay, he can just wheel you across the street. Makes things much easier."

"Easier on whom? What are you talking about?"

"Sister Elsie went to the cardiologist on a Monday, and she ended up staying in the hospital for two weeks."

I just shake my head.

"Sister Susie went to the cardiologist on a Tuesday, and she ended up on the psychiatric ward."

I say to myself, "This makes no sense."

"Come to think of it, Sister Susie did have a few screws missing. She was really nutty, especially when she forgot to take her meds. Last week she was in the choir stand with her wig turned inside out. I still don't see how she was able to keep that ugly wig on her head. I just know she forgot to take her medication. I bet it was Sister Willa's fault. Sister Willa is new to the Pastor's Aide Committee. The committee is responsible for calling the sick and the shut-ins for the Reverend. Sister Crouse puts Sister Susie's name on the list every Sunday, and beside her name she writes: 'Remind Sister Susie to take her meds or else she will go crazy.'"

I start to laugh.

"Just trying to make you feel better. Laughter is good."

"Thanks."

"Try not to worry, dear. It will all be okay. You are just going to have to learn to slow down and take it easy."

"Yeah, easier said than done. In my line of work as an obstetrician, it is not going to be easy," I think to myself.

"Let me know if I need to stop by the insurance office and see Brother Will while I am out. He cut back on his hours because he has been drinking. Tomorrow is payday. I know Brother Will is in the office, broke and sober. It's the best time for him to write up a policy. I will be on that side of town. I can pick up the papers for you to sign. It is no trouble, no trouble at all."

Chapter 2

Mercy General Hospital

I walk in the house and go straight to my room. I change clothes and immediately climb into bed. My head hurts, and all I want to do is sleep. I close my eyes.

My mind wanders back to my OB/GYN days at the General. I visualize the old on-call team, which consisted of an attending physician (the boss), chief resident (fourth-year resident), mid-level resident (second- or third-year resident), intern (basic scutt monkey—that was me), and a third- or fourth-year medical student. Some nights we had a visiting emergency medical services member or a student nurse.

My main job as the intern on the team was to manage the obstetrical triage area and facilitate all the normal, uncomplicated vaginal deliveries. I was also in charge of inserting the IV lines and drawing the blood work for the laboratory studies ordered on patients.

In my mind, I picture the face of Nurse Iris. She was a gray-haired lady with an imposing physique. She kept a stern look on her face and was the only nurse in the hospital who wore the old starched white uniform with the distinctive school's nursing cap.

Nurse Iris was in charge, and she had no problem letting everyone know that she was the *boss*. She was always serious, and her pursuit of excellence drove us all crazy. I very seldom saw Nurse Iris lose her temper. She only yelled when it was really serious. In all my years of medicine since, I have not worked with a smarter or more authoritative nurse. That is how the overall staff were at the General. The place brought the toughest and best out of everyone.

Whenever I worked with Nurse Iris, I obeyed all her commands. Yes, I was the queen of the Obstetrical Triage Area. In *theory*, I was in charge of admitting patients to the hospital. In *reality,* it was a different story. If Nurse Iris said to admit a patient to the hospital and send her to Labor and Delivery, then to Labor and Delivery the patient would go. If Nurse Iris said the patient was not in labor, home the patient would go.

When I was on-call with Nurse Iris, I cherished her advice. I was not going to take any chances with the lives of my patients. I knew my limitations and skills; actually, let's just say, I knew I had all the *limitations* and Nurse Iris had all the *skills*. Nurse Iris definitely had more experience than me. In my mind and everyone else's, Nurse Iris was the Obstetrical Triage "Boss."

I remember a lot of baby mama drama on one particular on-call shift. It was a full moon, and we got slammed. I'm not sure what the moon has to do with babies, but I do know one thing: on that particular day the patients kept walking in with all kinds of complaints. It was worse than the after-Christmas sale at the mall. We were flooded with patient walk-ins and patient drop-offs from the paramedics. There were no true obstetrical emergencies. The people who walked through the hospital doors arrived to escape from their own personal drama at home. They brought their *baby mama drama* to the General's Labor and Delivery, and I was quickly overwhelmed.

♦♦♦♦♦♦♦♦♦♦♦♦♦♦♦♦♦♦♦♦♦♦♦♦♦♦♦

Patient 1

A lady came in complaining of pain in her foot. She informed us that the pain had been there for ten days. When I examined her foot, I did not see a cut, redness, or any evidence of swelling. The patient screamed when she watched me examine her foot. When I distracted her, she forgot all about the pain and did not even flinch.

Nurse Iris quickly told me what to do, "Dr. Jones, send that crazy woman home with a prescription for Extra Strength Tylenol. She comes in here all the time trying to get drugs to sell. All she wants is some Percocet or something else with codeine. Percocet sells for five to ten dollars a pill on the black market. A patient can make two or three hundred bucks on one prescription of thirty Percocet tablets."

"You got it, Iris. Here are her discharge papers and a prescription for Extra Strength Tylenol."

The patient exclaimed, "Extra Strength Tylenol! What am I supposed to do with this?"

Nurse Iris replied, "You are instructed to take two tablets every six to eight hours as needed for pain. Do not take more than six tablets in a twenty-four-hour period. If the pain comes back, follow up with your obstetrician in the morning."

"If the pain comes back? It's not gone. I still have pain in my foot."

Nurse Iris handed the prescription to the patient.

The patient looked down at the prescription. "I got some of this stuff at home and it doesn't work," she said, "You could at least make it Tylenol #3, or something stronger with codeine. What am I supposed to do with this Extra Strength Tylenol prescription? I can't sell this Tylenol. Nobody wants to buy this stuff. They give away this cheap stuff at the clinic."

Nurse Iris and I stared at the patient.

"Oops, it's my foot. It's really hurting. Tylenol won't help. I need something for my foot. Extra Strength Tylenol is no good for my pain."

Nurse Iris replied firmly, "You get what the doctor ordered. You are discharged to leave. Don't forget to follow up with your Obstetrician. If your foot is still bothering you at your next scheduled doctor's appointment, let your doctor know and you can be examined again. Now go."

"Last time I was here, the doctor gave me something stronger to help calm my nerves. I need something for my nerves. You can at least give me something for my nerves?"

"You get what the doctor ordered. The doctor prescribed Extra Strength Tylenol."

"I don't want this Tylenol. I know my rights. I want to see another doctor. I want to see somebody else."

Now Nurse Iris became angry. "If you don't put on your clothes and leave, I will call hospital security and have you thrown out of here. I have other patients to see. Now go. I have women in labor to take care of who really need help. I will give you five minutes before I call hospital security," she exclaimed.

Nurse Iris then moved on to the next patient. The patient grabbed her things and stormed out of the obstetrical triage area.

"I am not coming back here. I will have my baby someplace else."

Nurse Iris and I gave each other the same look and said, "Goodbye and good luck with your delivery. We wish you well."

In our line of business, the patients who claim they don't want to come back to see us, always do. This hospital is the only trauma hospital in the inner city. When the patients do return, it is usually by ambulance and in an obstetrical emergency. They are the true baby mama dramas and usually they are disastrous. I don't wish that kind of drama on anybody—especially not on an unborn baby.

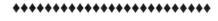

Patient 2

The next patient walked into the obstetrical triage area and complained that her knee had been hurting for days. She weighed 350 pounds and wanted a walking cane to help her get around. I examined her knee; there were no medical problems. She exhibited no tenderness and a good range of motion. I sent her home with a routine follow up with her obstetrical doctor and yes, Extra Strength Tylenol if she needed it for pain.

"Thank you doctor, can I have my cane now?"

"We don't have walking canes here," Nurse Iris explained, "This area is for obstetrical emergencies. You have to get a walking cane from your regular OB doctor."

"My regular doctor gave me a prescription for a walking cane, but my insurance company would not pay for it. I have trouble getting around. I have no money to purchase a cane. I need help. You see how hard it is for me to carry this baby and move around."

Nurse Iris replied, "You decided you would come to the hospital at 2:30 a.m. and try to get a walking cane from us? This area is for obstetrical emergencies only. We take care of patients in labor, patients who need to be admitted to the hospital, or patients who are about to die. You don't fit any of those descriptions. Here is your <u>Extra Strength Tylenol</u> prescription. You are discharged to go home. I suggest you leave. And don't forget to follow-up with your regular obstetrician."

The patient threw the Extra Strength Tylenol prescription in Nurse Iris' face: "That is what you can do with your attitude and this Tylenol prescription," she yelled.

Nurse Iris, showing much restraint, replied, "If you don't get out of here, I will call the hospital security."

The patient hobbled out the door muttering, "If I had a walking cane I would beat you with it. I would take the walking cane and wrap it around your neck. I would hit you so hard that you would see glory."

"That's why you get no walking cane. Now get to stepping or, in your case, get to hobbling. Return to the hospital only if you have contractions, break your bag of water, start to have vaginal bleeding, or you don't feel your baby moving. Now go. Get out of here. And follow up with your regular obstetrician."

◆◆◆◆◆◆◆◆◆◆◆◆◆◆◆◆◆◆◆◆◆◆◆◆◆◆◆

Patient 3

The next patient came to the obstetrical triage area complaining of a dry cough. She had a history of smoking six packs of cigarettes per day. She denied having fever, chills, or a sore throat. I talked to her about smoking cessation but my words fell on deaf ears. She was not interested in anything I had to say.

"I need some Robitussin with codeine and some of those Tussalin Pearls," she informed me.

I examined the patient's throat. No redness, no swelling, no tenderness, and no fever.

Nurse Iris said, "Here we go again. This patient is just seeking drugs. She has not coughed since she walked through the triage doors."

"What are Tussalin Pearls?" I asked Nurse Iris.

"They are Tussionex[3] capsules, otherwise known as Tussalin Pearles. They contain hydrocodone and the antihistamine chlorpheniramine. They were once used to give medication to soldiers out in the field so they would not give away their position because of a cough. Now the drug addicts get the medication and melt the capsules down. They then inject the medication into their veins. I am told they get a pretty nice high. They say that the effect is somewhere between heroin and crack cocaine. Apparently, the medication is really cheap and easy to find on the black market."

"Dr. Jones, you should never prescribe Tussionex capsules. The Drug Enforcement Agency (DEA) knows all about the illegal use of Tussionex. If you prescribe a lot of those capsules, the DEA will be all over you. You definitely don't need that headache. The DEA can be relentless. They have cost some doctors their careers. Your career is just starting."

"Thanks Nurse Iris; that is good information to know."

Nurse Iris turned to the patient: "You are discharged to go. Take your <u>Extra Strength Tylenol</u> prescription and go home. Drink plenty of fluids and return only if you have contractions, break your bag of water, start to have vaginal bleeding, or you don't feel your baby moving."

"I don't want a Tylenol prescription. I want something for my cough. I need some Robitussin with codeine, and I want some Tussalin Pearls."

"You get what the doctor prescribes for you. You are discharged to leave. Take this Extra Strength Tylenol prescription and follow-up with your obstetrician. Now go. Get out of here."

◆◆◆◆◆◆◆◆◆◆◆◆◆◆◆◆◆◆◆◆◆◆◆◆◆◆◆

Patient 4

The next patient came in and complained that she had been unable to sleep for six days. It was 3:00 a.m. and obstetrical triage area was overflowing with non-laboring patients. Everybody wanted a prescription for something. I felt like a drug pusher—just one that was not getting paid.

Nurse Iris handed the patient a prescription for Tylenol PM: "This medication will help you sleep, and it will not harm the baby."

"I can get this over the counter. I need something stronger to help me sleep." "Have you taken Tylenol PM before?"

"No, but my sister takes the medicine that comes on television for sleep. What is the name of that stuff? I remember, it is called Ambien. I need some Ambien, 12.5 mg, for sleep—and I don't want no generic stuff."

Nurse Iris responded immediately, "Now we get down to the real truth. You even know the strength of the medication is Ambien 12.5 mg. The doctor prescribed Tylenol PM; that is what you get. Here is your prescription. You are now discharged to go home."

"That stuff is no good. Tylenol PM is over the counter."

"If you run out of medication, you don't have to come back here for a refill. You can get it over the counter. You are discharged to leave. Follow up with your regular obstetrician, or call the clinic in the morning to make an appointment. Here is the clinic number. Drink plenty of fluids and return only if you have contractions, break your bag of water, start to have vaginal bleeding, or you don't feel your baby moving."

The patient left with a very bad attitude. She verbalized her unhappiness to everyone in the waiting area. "They gave me some Tylenol PM. What am I supposed to do with this stuff? They could have at least given me some pills."

I overheard the conversation and turned to Nurse Iris. "What do people think? Do they think we just hand out free medication here?"

"It's sad but true; some people think that we are a free service center that provides free medication and free treatment."

At 4:25 a.m., the staff were exhausted and grumpy, and we were all operating on fumes. I briefly laid my head on the nurses' station counter. Nurse Iris walked over to me.

"Dr. Jones it is now 4:30 a.m., and no one in the obstetrical triage area is in real labor. Why don't you go to the on-call room and take a quick nap? I will call you at 5:30 a.m. and wake you up.

"Thanks, Iris, that's a great idea."

♦♦♦♦♦♦♦♦♦♦♦♦♦♦♦♦♦♦♦♦♦♦♦♦♦♦♦

I staggered down the hall in a daze and located the on-call room. The door was locked. The only way to open the door was with a plastic card. I had forgotten to get a plastic card when I was in triage. I managed to walk back into the obstetrical triage area.

"Iris I can't get into the on-call room. Can I have a blank patient identification card?"

The key to the call room had been missing for about five years. I am sure that one of the former residents forgot to return it and the department was too cheap to purchase a new one. In any event, we were the ones to suffer. The only way to open the on-call room door was with a plastic patient identification card. My first skill in training as an intern was the art of breaking into the on-call room. This skill served me well.

Nurse Iris handed me a plastic card.

"Here Dr. Jones, you better take two just in case you lose this one. I will give you a call at 5:30 a.m."

"Thanks, Iris."

I took the cards and then stumbled back to the on-call room. I opened the door with the plastic card, walked into the room and sat on the edge of the bed. I stared at the ceiling in a trance. I pulled off my clogs and began to massage my legs. My feet were swollen. I couldn't believe my ankles were swollen, too. This could not be happening. My legs never swelled. My mind started to race with a differential diagnosis of swelling feet, ankles, and legs. "I am too young for lower extremity swelling. This is not good. I am too young," I thought.

I began my differential diagnosis with pathological conditions—poor circulation, heart problems, kidney problems, or a blood clot. I begin to ponder. I came to my senses. There is nothing pathologic about this condition. This lower extremity problem is just physiologic. It originates from standing on my poor, aching legs too long. My legs have taken a beating. Nothing should be upright for more than twenty hours. I released a sigh of relief. Gravity had pulled all my blood from my brain. The blood was now in my legs.

Looking down at my feet I said to myself, "The proof is in the swelling."

I massaged my ankles and then propped them up on a pillow and closed my eyes. I drifted off to sleep and started dreaming instantly. In my dream, I was far away from baby mama drama on Labor and Delivery in the OB triage area. I could no longer hear people say: "This hurts—That hurts—I want—I need." Instead, I saw the sun, the sand and the beach. I smelled the salt in the air. It was so inviting. I continued to dream.

The pager went off two separate times, but I didn't hear the beeps. I was deep in my fantasy sleep, and my body did not want to be disturbed. In those days the pagers we carried were voice-activated. The page would start with a loud beep. Following the beep, the voice message would be relayed. The problem with the voice-activated system was that many of the messages could not be heard over the static. If the beep was missed, there was no way to tell who called or the intention of the message. The only hope was to wait for the page to come again. Digital pagers are so much better. Technology is definitely one giant leap for mankind; or, in our case, one giant leap for patient care.

Realizing I must have been sleeping, Nurse Iris told the clerk to call the phone in the on-call room. The phone rang. I grabbed my pager, thinking that the noise was emitting from there. I was in a total daze, and felt as though my mind was playing tricks on me. I was in that zone between conscious awareness and the afterlife. I was still hanging out at the beach with its warm sand, the beautiful sky, and the inviting water.

The phone stopped and then started again. By now I had come to my senses sufficiently to realize that it was the phone ringing. I looked at the clock. It was 5:01 a.m. I picked up the phone. It was Nurse Iris: "Dr. Jones come quickly; we have a delivery in Labor Room 3."

I hung up the phone and put my swollen feet back into my shoes. I grabbed my pager and dashed out the door.

Chapter 3

Breech Delivery

I walked into Labor Room 3.
The patient was out of control. All she did was yell, cuss, and swear… and then swear, cuss, and yell some more. Yes, that was Mrs. Felicia Ferdinane Fagon up close and in person. She smelled like a distillery and had a temperament to match.

I walked to her bedside and looked down. On my initial examination, I saw the baby's butt coming through the birth canal (breech). My eyes opened wide, and my tongue stuck to the roof of my mouth. My throat felt dry, and I could not swallow. I squinted, hoping my eyes were deceiving me. I looked again—no such luck. The baby's butt was coming out first.

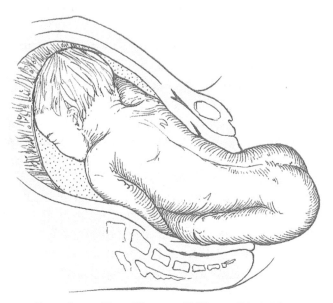

Breech position. (Source: Williams Obstetrics 22nd Edition, 2005, page 574).[4]

I was paralyzed with fear for an instant. I regained my composure and looked again. I wanted to have my facts correct to give a report to my backup superior. I looked down and saw a pool of blood dripping on the floor. I got scared. I got really… really… really… scared.

My heart dropped, and my breathing slowed. The sound of blood splashing got louder and louder. I heard every drop of blood hit the floor. Since my eyes were playing tricks on me, and my ears were no help, I turned all my attention to my head. I thought: "If I can just get some oxygen to my brain, then I can think. I can figure out what to do. I need to think." I took a deep breath. The problem with deep breathing was that my sense of smell took over, and the stench was beyond words. Mrs. Fagon was sitting in a pool of bodily waste, and the smell was terrible.

Chills are going down my spine now as I recall today the mental picture of Mrs. Fagon. Her feet appeared to have been pulled through a mud bank of wild onions and something else that had left behind a dark red and green stain, while her legs resembled the back end of an elephant with skin as tough as rawhide. Her breasts touched her belly button and looked like two over-the-hill Trojan warriors. The two worn-out saddle bags just flapping in the breeze were her arms. Each strand of her hair was waging its own personal battle, and not one of them was winning.

I can remember her total lack of hygiene, as well. Her breath smelled of old garlic mixed with something so pungent that I couldn't even recognize it. It was obvious that her entire exterior had seen no water, friend or foe, in at least two weeks. Her bottom was wedged into a large pile of stool mixed with old urine, and she smelled of toxic waste. I dared not speculate the last time she saw soap or anything resembling a cleaning solution. In addition, her mouth was spewing out one cuss after another: abusive, vulgar obscenities. Overall, Mrs. Fagon was out of control. She looked rough, talked tough, and was just plain mean.

I tried hard to hold my breath, but it was no use. I began to gasp for air. I opened my mouth and tried to speak. With a squeaky tone, I managed to say, "Nurse Iris, I need help. I really need some help. I don't know how to deliver a butt-baby… I mean a breech baby."

Nurse Iris answered, "Attending Physician Dr. Smith is in the labor room next door; Chief Resident Michael Morris is in labor Room 6; and the second-year resident, Priscilla Coleman, is downstairs, admitting a patient from the Emergency Room. You have no backup. You're on your own. You're the doctor in charge in this room."

"No one but me?"

I tried to swallow, but my throat was too dry. Terror gripped me. I felt like I had been hit by a lightning bolt, the jolt of which started in my feet and traveled up to my head. I felt lightheaded. I was terrified. I was unprepared, and it showed.

"No direct doctor supervision?" I thought, "I'm only an intern. I just got out of med school six weeks ago! This lady needs a real doctor. This lady needs somebody who knows how to deliver a butt-baby."

I began to panic. My thoughts ran rampant: *I am scared for myself. I am frightened for Mrs. Fagon. I am really terrified for this baby. This is not good.* I tried to relieve my anxieties with a pep talk.

I remember my grandmother's wisdom. "Seek God's will in all you do, and he will show you which path to take" (Proverbs 3:6).[5]

I said to myself, "God help me. Show me what to do. If you say run out of this room, I'm with you. If you tell me to go, then we are both out of here." I waited for a reply. What was I thinking? I could not leave the scene. I had to stay and help.

Talk about OJT (On the Job Training) at the General. That is how it was back in those days. It was either sink or swim. So I learned to do the doggy paddle and roll with the punches. Trust me, it was not easy.

Delivering a breech baby through the vaginal canal is very dangerous. The biggest risk to the baby is head entrapment. The human body is amazing. The cervix will dilate to accommodate whatever it first encounters. Normally that is the head, which is the largest part of the body. The cervix will dilate to accommodate the head then the rest of the body just slips out nicely. In the case of a breech baby, the cervix will dilate enough for whatever it sees first (butt or legs). Since the head is larger than the legs, the head can get stuck and cause head entrapment, which is an obstetrical nightmare that can kill a baby quickly.

The possibility of head entrapment is especially risky for first-time mothers. In the case of first-time mothers, most doctors will perform a cesarean section and deliver the baby safely through the abdomen.

I reminded myself, "I may not know much about breech deliveries, but I do know something about delivering normal babies."

I started with a normal delivery, and from there I tried hard to remember the rules for delivering a breech. There are seven rules, and I could only remember four. I hoped the four rules I remembered were the most important ones, and that the three I had forgotten would not cause the baby too much harm.

What was I thinking? If someone came up with seven rules, they must all be important. I was definitely in the land of "for better or worse," and this baby was paying the price of my lack of knowledge and limited skill. Things were looking grim but, through it all, I continued to shake and pray.

The rules I remembered for vaginal breech delivery:

Rule Number 1 = Delivery person with experience.
Rule Number 2 = Calculate baby's age and weight.
Rule Number 3 = Is the birth canal big enough?
Rule Number 4 = Is the delivery team available for surgery?

<u>Rule number 1</u> is to have a delivery person with some experience. This is a no-brainer. I'm an intern. I just got out of medical school six weeks ago. I said to myself: "Experienced operator." Mrs. Fagon really needed someone who had at least seen a breech delivery before. The closest I had come to a breech delivery was looking at the pictures in my obstetrical textbooks.

I thought, "What will happen if this baby gets into trouble and the mother needs an emergency cesarean delivery? At this stage in my training, I'm not qualified to perform a breech extraction or surgery. I just graduated from medical school six weeks ago, and I can barely do a normal, uncomplicated vaginal delivery."

Poor, poor, Mrs. Fagon.

It is sad when you get the first rule wrong. It shakes you up and can destroy any confidence you have to continue. And trust me, I was already scared and did not need any further shaking. I deleted Rule Number 1 from my mental checklist.

Rule number 2 is to know the baby's age and weight. Gestational age is determined by knowing the mother's last menstrual period or by performing an ultrasound examination to measure the baby's head, abdomen, and thigh bone.

I looked at Mrs. Fagon. It was too late for the ultrasound. I took a deep breath and opened my mouth to speak: "Ma'am, do you know the first day of your last menstrual period?"

She replied: "I have no *%#* clue. Get this *%#* kid out of me."

Nurse Iris had been doing this much longer than me. I was sure that she knew the age and weight of the baby just by looking at Mrs. Fagon.

I turned to Nurse Iris: "Iris, what's the gestational age of this baby?"

"Mrs. Fagon is a little chubby."

Mrs. Fagon didn't appreciate that comment, "Who you calling fat? You big-headed *%#* pork chop."

Nurse Iris ignored Mrs. Fagon's outburst. She continued, "By the size of Mrs. Fagon's belly, I would say she is about eight months pregnant. This baby is possibly eight-to-ten weeks premature."

In my mind, Nurse Iris' *possibly* was better than my *no clue*.

"Iris, what's the baby's weight?"

"I would say around 2,000 grams."

"How many *%#* pounds is that?" Mrs. Fagon asked.

I thought to myself: "Good question, Mrs. Fagon. I want to know this answer too." I knew there are 454 grams in one pound but, without a calculator, my processor ran slow.

Nurse Iris replied: "Four pounds and four ounces or somewhere close."

"That sounds small."

"It is small. Your baby is premature and breech."

"Breech! Nurse, you mean it's a butt-baby?"

"Yes, Mrs. Fagon, the baby is breech and at risk of birth trauma if you don't cooperate."

According to Nurse Iris, the age of the baby was eight months and the weight was 4 pounds and some change. I checked off Rule Number 2 from my mental checklist.

Rule Number 3 is to know whether the mother's birth canal is large enough to deliver the baby. I recalled a lecture on clinical assessment of the pelvis that I had attended a week earlier. I was a post-call zombie during the lecture and had pretty much slept through everything. However, I vaguely remembered something about measuring the pelvic inlet, pelvic outlet, and assessing the mid pelvis. Fortunately for me, this was Mrs.

Fagon's sixth baby number; as such, five other babies had all come out of this birth canal. This baby was premature, so it should just fall out. The birth canal of Mrs. Fagon was definitely big enough. I checked off Rule Number 3 from my mental checklist.

<u>Rule Number 4</u> is to have the delivery team available for surgery. I looked around the room. Mrs. Fagon needed someone who could perform an emergency cesarean delivery if she got into trouble. I was no help to Mrs. Fagon; I was not qualified to perform surgery on anybody. I deleted Rule Number 4 from my mental checklist and reviewed my answers.

Rules (of those I remembered) for vaginal breech delivery

Rule Number 1 = Delivery person with experience. **No**
Rule Number 2 = Calculate baby age and weight. **Yes**
Rule Number 3 = Is birth canal big enough? **Yes**
Rule Number 4 = Is the delivery team available for surgery? **No**

I thought, "Out of four rules that I have remembered, I had two rules that I was sure were correct. I could not remember Rule 5, Rule 6, or Rule 7. In reality, the total count was two out of seven. Those were not good odds for anything. Definitely not good in a life-or-death situation." For Mrs. Fagon and the baby's sake, I hoped that two out of seven were good enough, because that was all I had to offer.

Nurse Iris, sensing my anxiety, said, "The only available help for Mrs. Fagon are you and the medical student Berney Poindexter."

I looked at Nurse Iris, "You have got to be kidding. This lady needs a real doctor. She needs more than me and a scared, useless medical student."

Medical Student Berney was certainly no help. Berney was a paramedic, and he claimed to have worked in the field for over ten years. When I asked Berney to tell me the number of babies he delivered, he said none. Not one baby. I believed Berney because he absolutely hated obstetrics. That's how it works. You either love obstetrics or you want no part of it. Medical Student Berney made it abundantly clear that he wanted no part in the delivery of babies. He didn't care for the sound of screaming mothers or out-of-control crying babies. I was certain there would be no plans for labor and delivery in Berney's future.

With Berney as my only choice for help, I knew I was on my own. The frightening truth began to set in. I had to deliver this baby. It was just me and Nurse Iris. I continued to shake.

"Okay, Iris, what do I do?"

Mrs. Fagon screamed, "What do you do? You get this *%#* butt-baby out of me! That is what you *%#* do! You get this butt-baby out of me!"

I shook so hard that I tore a hole in my glove. Nurse Iris saw my unsteady hands and walked to the cabinet where the supplies were kept.

"Dr. Jones, you have a latex allergy. Are Biogel gloves okay? They are supposed to be latex-free."

I managed to say in a whisper, "Biogels are fine."

My tremor began to get worst. Nurse Iris then handed me a pair of gloves.

Mrs. Fagon screamed, "You've gotta be kidding me. That doctor can't even put her hand in a glove. How the *%#* is she gonna catch my butt-baby?"

Nurse Iris ignored her, "Calm down, Dr. Jones. It'll be okay. Just calm down."

I tried really hard to talk myself into a calm and assertive mode, but the shaking was uncontrollable. Beads of sweat flooded my forehead. They trickled into my eyes and blinded my vision. Perspiration collected on my face shield. It was difficult to breathe.

Nurse Iris repeated, "Calm down, Dr. Jones. This is baby number six, and it is a small, premature baby. Best guess, the baby is about eight weeks early. Calm down, I'll talk you through the delivery."

I said to myself, "Something is wrong with this tiny baby. Something is keeping this baby from falling out, and I don't know what it is. Nurse Iris is right, this is baby number six. This kid should just fall out." I tried really hard to calm down, but the sweat continued to run into my eyes. My breathing was labored, and everyone in the room could hear me struggle. Nurse Iris patted my forehead and wiped the sweat.

"Thank you Iris, now I can see."

Mrs. Fagon shrieked, "I'm glad you can see, but it sounds to me that you can't *%#* breathe. How are you gonna catch my butt-baby when you can't breathe?"

My entire head was congested, and it was obvious that everyone in the room could hear me struggling. I took a deep breath.

I reminded myself, "Breathe, Chandra, breathe. Be calm and assertive and breathe."

Mrs. Fagon was unrelenting, "You better breathe first. Then get this *%#*___ butt-baby out of me?"

Nurse Iris: "Dr. Jones, breathe slowly and calm down."

Mrs. Fagon looked at Nurse Iris, and said, "Nurse, you told her to *%#*___ breathe and calm down. Isn't that what you're supposed to be telling me to do? I am the one having a *%#* butt-baby. Get this *%#* butt-baby out of me."

I looked at Nurse Iris. The patient was right, but this was not the time for an interrogation.

I reminded myself, "Breathe, calm down, I can do this."

Mrs. Fagon carried on: "Did you say talk her through the *%#* delivery? I want a real doctor. I don't want no *%#* trainee. I know my *%#* rights. Get me a real doctor, or I'll sue everybody in this place. I'll sue all of you. I tell you, I'll sue. I know my *%#* rights."

"Calm down Mrs. Fagon and help us deliver this little premature baby," Nurse Iris pleaded

"Give me some *%#* drugs. Get me a real *%#* doctor. I'm not a *%#* guinea pig. I'm not here for *%#* practice. Get me a real *%#* doctor. I want some *%#* drugs, now. I tell you, I'll sue you and everyone in the hospital. When I get done with this place, it'll be called Fagon South Central."

Medical Student Berney walked in and surveyed the room. He saw blood covering the bed and dripping on the floor. From the corner of my eye, I saw Berney ease over to the corner and hug the wall.

Berney was really something. He was 6'2", weighed 325 pounds, and looked like a defensive tackler who played in the National Football League. It was a good thing that he was hugging the wall. If he fell and hit one of us, somebody could have gotten seriously injured.

I had once seen a medical student pass out in the operating room during my medical school days. The student was immediately taken to the emergency room where he was diagnosed as having a mild concussion. He never lived down the experience. After passing out in the operating room, the staff started calling him Dropsy.

I saw Dropsy at the OB/GYN National Conference last year. He is now in charge of the obstetrical division at the prestigious Vanderbilt Hospital. Everybody has a story. Dropsy sure has a good one.

Nurse Iris instructed, "Dr. Jones, put your hands around the baby's legs and gently pull."

Mrs. Fagon parroted, "Pull, *%#*, pull! All you have to do is pull."

Nurse Iris spoke into the speaker located on the bed rail, "We need the pediatricians. Call the NICU (Neonatal Intensive Care Unit). Tell them they're getting an admission. Tell the team to get here stat."

I placed my hands gently on the baby's legs and gave a slight pull.

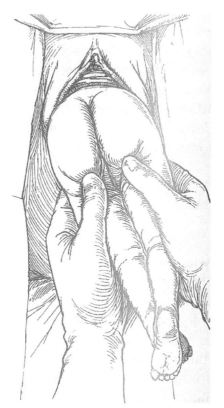

Breech delivery (Source: *Williams Obstetrics* 22nd Edition, 2005, 576).[4]

I was so scared that I was going to bruise the legs. What was I thinking? The legs were already blue. Even if I did grab the legs too tightly, we would never be able to tell if what I did caused the injury. This baby was already banged and bruised up.

All progress soon stopped. I started to panic.

"Iris, nothing is happening. The baby just stopped moving."

"What do you mean nothing's happening?" Asked Mrs. Fagon, "Just pull the *%#* butt-baby out. Just pull, *%#*, pull. Get this butt-baby out of me." Nurse Iris commanded, "Mrs. Fagon, calm down."

"Calm down my foot. I'm getting outta this place. I'm going someplace where I can get some *%#* help. You dumb *%#* don't know what you're doing."

Mrs. Fagon tried to get out of the bed. It became a struggle to hold her down. In the middle of all the pandemonium, Mrs. Fagon kicked Student Nurse Melissa in the chest. Melissa dropped Mrs. Fagon's leg, grabbed her chest, and started to scream. Imagine the scene. I had a hysterical mother in Mrs. Fagon, a screaming student nurse, a no-help medical student, and a motionless baby. But I also had Commando Nurse Iris.

I raised my eyes and looked at Nurse Iris for help. Nurse Iris used her infantry commando voice, "Melissa, go to the nursing station and send Rachel in. Berney get over here. Melissa, move; Berney, move... now!"

Then she turned her attention to Mrs. Fagon. "Mrs. Fagon, we need you to cooperate. Calm yourself down for the sake of this baby. Take a deep breath and push this tiny baby out. Stop acting like you've never done this before. You can do this. This is baby number six. I know you can do this. Now control yourself and start pushing."

Mrs. Fagon shook her head violently, "I want some *%#* drugs. Get me some morphine."

Nurse Iris gave orders. "Berney, get over here and grab the back of Mrs. Fagon's leg. Rachel, support the back of Mrs. Fagon's neck. That way she won't have a headache when all this is over."

"A headache? That is the least of my worries!" shouted Mrs. Fagon, "I want some *%#* drugs, and I don't want no generic stuff. Get me some real drugs!" "Berney, move. I mean move now."

"Who me?"

"Yes you, I am talking to you. Get over here, and hold up Mrs. Fagon's leg."

Medical Student Berney remained motionless. It was hard to tell if he was actually breathing.

Nurse Iris used her infantry commando voice once again, "Berney now! Move! I mean move!"

Medical Student Berney started to walk in slow motion towards the bedside. Meanwhile, Nurse Iris continued to issue orders: "Rachel, support the back of Mrs. Fagon's neck, and put her chin to her chest." Student Nurse Rachel reached for the back of Mrs. Fagon's neck, but Mrs. Fagon screamed, "If you touch me I'll punch you. Don't put your filthy *%#* hands on me. I'll sue. I tell you I'll sue. If you put your filthy hands on me, I'll sue."

I thought, "The only thing in here that's filthy and out-of-control is the mouth of this lady. Since I have been in this room, all she has done is yell, cuss, and swear."

The door to the delivery room opened. It was Dr. Mark Chase and the Neonatology team. Dr. Chase was the chief neonatologist. If anyone could save a baby, it was definitely Dr. Chase. Miracles happened when Dr. Chase walked into a room. I was really glad that he had walked into this one. At least something was starting to go right. He asked, "What do we have here?"

Nurse Iris answered, "Patient about eight weeks premature came in completely dilated. Baby is breech. Heart tones are now starting to fall. Don't have any other history on the mother."

The normal heart rate for a fetus is 120-160 beats per minute. As Dr. Chase and his staff assembled the resuscitation equipment on the baby warmer, the heart rate fell to the 90s. That was not good.

"How long have the baby's heart tones been down?"

Nurse Iris replied, "Not long. The heart tones go down to the 90s with each contraction, but they go back to normal when the contraction is over. So far, the baby is handling it well. No fetal distress yet."

"That is good news," I thought, "At least this baby was hanging in there." Normal heart tones following a uterine contraction mean that the blood flow through the umbilical cord is as expected. Good blood flow means good oxygen for the fetus and no fetal distress.

Dr. Chase asked, "Any drugs on board that we need to know about?"

Dr. Chase needed to know if the mother had received any narcotics. If Mrs. Fagon had narcotics in her system, the baby could have difficulty breathing when it was delivered. If narcotics were in her system, they could be neutralized by giving the baby a drug called Naloxone. Naloxone is an antidote for morphine and other narcotic drugs.

Nurse Iris reported, "Not from our end. No narcotics from us. We didn't have enough time to run a drug screen. Better get it from your end."

Mrs. Fagon interrupted, "I want some drugs, but these stingy *%#* won't give them to me! Help me Doc, I need some drugs!"

Nurse Iris, ignoring Mrs. Fagon's request for drugs, said, "Mrs. Fagon, put your chin to your chest and push. Your baby's heart rate is dropping."

The heart rate was in the mid-60s, and it was not going back up to the normal range.

"If you don't push your baby is going to die. Push, Mrs. Fagon. Give it all you got, and push this little baby out."

Nurse Iris started the count. I continued to pull on the legs, and the baby began to inch down slowly.

"Iris, the baby is starting to move."

Nurse Iris said, encouragingly, "Good Dr. Jones, just keep up the slow gentle traction."

The movement stopped when I reached the baby's shoulders. I looked at the fetal heart rate. It was back to normal.

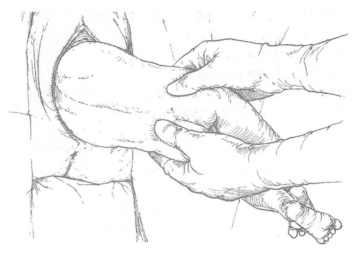

Delivering the shoulders (Source: *Williams Obstetrics, 22nd Edition*, 2005, 576).[4]

"Iris, the baby is not moving. I can't pull the baby out."

I could feel everyone's eyes in the room burning a hole through me. I tried to keep my composure, but I knew panic was written all over my face. I felt the sweat running down my back. I believed time was standing still. At least that was what I was hoping.

At that point, Nurse Iris instructed, "Turn the baby clockwise. Slip your hand under the back of the baby's shoulder. Follow the shoulder to the arm."

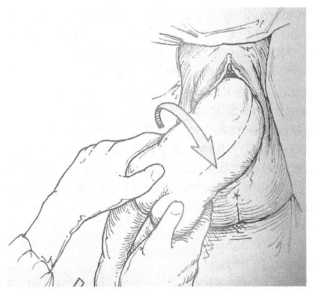

Rotating the baby (Source: *Williams Obstetrics, 22nd Edition*, 2005, 576).[4]

"Okay, now what?"
"Pull the arm across the chest. Don't pull too hard. You don't want to damage the arm."

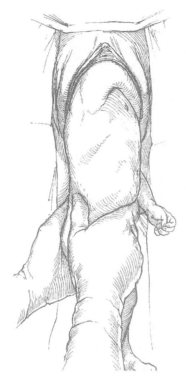

Arm across the chest (Source: *Williams Obstetrics*, 22nd Edition, 2005, 577).[4]

Mrs. Fagon once again spoke up, "Nurse, I heard you. You told her not to damage my baby. You better not damage my baby. My third child has a frozen arm. You better not hurt this baby. I'll sue. I'll *%#* sue."

Nurse Iris remained calm, "Calm down Mrs. Fagon. Dr. Jones is not going to damage your baby's arm."

"She better not hurt my baby. My baby better not get a frozen arm."

Student Nurse Rachel, now composed, whispered, "What is a frozen arm?"

Nurse Iris answered, "It's a brachial plexus injury."

Student Nurse Rachel commented, "Sounds bad."

I said to myself, "It is bad, and all this chit-chat is not helping me concentrate."

Mrs. Fagon again screamed, "Don't you give my baby a frozen arm. I'll sue you and this *%#* hospital. If you damage my baby, I'll sue. I'll name this place Fagon South Central."

I said to myself, "Like I don't have enough problems, now I have to listen to this." I refocused my attention on the instructions from Nurse Iris.

"Okay, Iris, what's next?"

Mrs. Fagon shrieked, "You still don't know what you're *%#* doing. Get this butt-baby out of me. That's what you do. Pull this butt-baby out of me. All you have to do is pull. Pull, *%#*, pull!"

Ignoring her rant, Nurse Iris said, "Now turn the baby the other way and deliver the other arm."

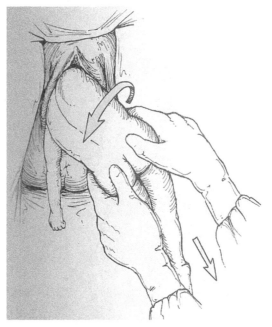

Delivering the second arm (Source: *Williams Obstetrics*, 22nd Edition, 2005, 575).[4]

Both arms were now delivered. I gave a slight pull, but the baby was stuck.

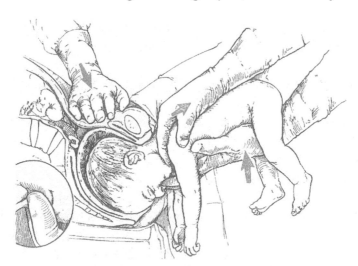

Preparing to deliver the head (Source: *Williams Obstetrics*, 22nd Edition, 2005, 578).[4]

Breech Delivery

"Iris, the head won't come out. It's stuck."

"What do you mean my baby is stuck? Get it outta me. Get it the *%#* outta me! I want this *%#* over."

At least this is the first thing that we both agreed on. We both wanted this baby mama drama to be over. "I'm definitely with you, Mrs. Fagon. I believe I want this delivery over much more than you do. I want freedom from you and this room," I thought.

Nurse Iris gently said, "Mrs. Fagon, stop pushing for a minute."

"First you say *%#* push. Then you say *%#* don't push. Would you make up your *%#* mind? Nurse, do you know what you're *%#* doing? Looks like I got all *%#* trainees in this room. Someone get me a real *%#*___ doctor and a real nurse. I want somebody in here who knows what the *%#* is going on. I want somebody in here who knows how to deliver a butt-baby. These *%#* fools don't know what they are doing."

Nurse Iris remained calm, "Mrs. Fagon, calm down and help this baby."

I thought, "Mrs. Fagon, shut up and help this baby."

Nurse Iris then pressed on Mrs. Fagon's pubic bone.

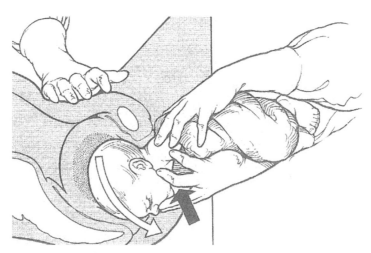

Delivering the head (Source: *Obstetrics—Normal and Problem Pregnancies*, 4th Edition, 2002, 486).[7]

Nurse Iris told me, "Dr. Jones, pull."

She then turned to Mrs. Fagon: "Mrs. Fagon, push as hard as you can; you can do this. If you don't push, your baby might not make it. *Push, Mrs. Fagon, Push.*"

Chanting started throughout the room: *"Push, Mrs. Fagon, Push."*

Mrs. Fagon held her breath. She put her chin to her chest and grabbed her legs. She bit her lip and gave a big push. The baby slowly inched out. I looked at the baby's chest to find signs of life. The entire body was bruised and it did not look good. I quickly clamped and cut the cord. I handed the baby to Dr. Chase. If anyone could bring this little baby back to life it was Dr. Chase. This was a time that we all needed a miracle.

The placenta soon delivered, and the drama was over.

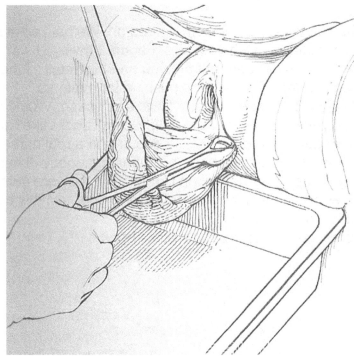

Delivering the placenta (Source: *Williams Obstetrics*, 22nd Edition, 2005, 576).[4]

I continued to massage Mrs. Fagon's uterus, thinking, "I have to contract the uterus and slow down the bleeding. If I don't slow the bleeding down, Mrs. Fagon will be in trouble."

"Doc, Doc! That hurts. You don't have to rub so *%#* hard. My belly is sore. I just *%#* had a baby. Stop mashing on my belly."

"Mrs. Fagon, you lost a lot of blood. I have to massage your uterus to help slow down the bleeding. If you continue to bleed, you will need a blood transfusion."

Mrs. Fagon continued her stream of abuse, "You aren't giving me no *%#*___ blood transfusion. I mean it, Doc. I don't want no *%#* blood transfusion." Nurse Iris asked me, "How is the bleeding? Is the uterus firm?"

"Yes, Iris, the uterus is starting to contract. The bleeding has slowed down. I think Mrs. Fagon will be all right."

"It is about time you had something good to *%#* say."

What I really wanted to say was, "My opinion is that I wish this woman would have delivered at another hospital. Any place with more breech experience would have been just fine. For that matter, she might have done better delivering this baby in the ambulance with the paramedics."

I looked over at Berney, "On second thought, maybe not."

Mrs. Fagon stared at me, "Look at her, she is over there *%#* shaking. I sure hope my baby is all right, and you didn't *%#* shake him all over the place. My baby better not have that *%#* shaken baby syndrome. I don't hear my baby. Doc, what's going on with my baby? I want to see my baby."

Once again, I thought, "I have got to get out of this room. This woman is driving me nuts. I need to get out of here and clear my head."

Nurse Iris, sensing my anxiety, said, "You did good, Dr. Jones. You did a good job for your first breech delivery."

"I heard you, nurse, you said that was her first butt-baby delivery. I knew she was a *%#* trainee. I knew that she didn't know what the *%#* she was doing. I knew she didn't know how to deliver a butt-baby."

"Calm down, Mrs. Fagon," Iris said.

"Calm down my foot. My baby better not have that *%#* shaken baby syndrome, or I will own this hospital. I tell you this place will be called Fagon South Central."

The baby began to make a little whimpering sound. This was the first sound of this baby's life. There was hope. We had all just witnessed a miracle.

Dr. Chase said, "I want to take the baby to the NICU (Neonatal Intensive Care Unit) to keep an eye on him."

"Give me my *%#* baby. I want to see my baby."

Dr. Chase wrapped the baby in a blanket and handed him to Mrs. Fagon.

Dr. Chase said, "He is a little one, and he has taken a beating. Other than his bumps and bruises, he should be alright."

"He better be *%#* alright. He just better be okay. If my baby does not grow up to be as smart and rich as Bill Gates, then I will own this place. I'll sue, and everybody in here will end up jobless and collecting food stamps."

She then looked over at me.

"This baby better be a *%#* rich genius."

"I bet nobody in her family is rich or a genius. She is a character and is trying to milk this delivery for all it is worth," I thought, but I continued to bite my lip.

Mrs. Fagon continued, "…And he better not have no *%#* shaken baby syndrome."

"It sure does take all kinds to make the world go round. This woman is really out there," I thought.

My Attending, Dr. Smith, entered the room. The room looked like a war zone. Blood was on the bedsheets, the floor, and all over me.

"Looks like you had your hands full. Any problems?" Dr. Smith asked.

"Any problems? It was baby mama drama at its worst. The baby was breech. The mother was hysterical. Student Nurse Melissa got kicked in the chest. Medical Student Berney was useless and absolutely no help. And the clincher was that I didn't know what I was doing… Nurse Iris rescued us all," I thought to myself.

Dr. Smith looked at Nurse Iris, "Any problems?"

I held my breath and waited. I knew Nurse Iris was going to tell Dr. Smith how terrified I was. I had no confidence and no clue. Most importantly, it had been Nurse Iris who had taken control and saved the day. I just happened to be standing in the room, sucking up air, and following directions.

Nurse Iris replied, "No problems. Dr. Jones did a good job delivering the breech baby." I thought I was hearing things, but I didn't want to question fate.

Dr. Smith was surprised, "Dr. Jones delivered what?"

"The baby was breech, and Dr. Jones did a good job. I don't think any other resident could have done better."

Nurse Iris then looked over at me and gave me a slight wink and a smile. She was really putting on a show for Dr. Smith, and I was so thankful.

"That's good, Dr. Jones," said Dr. Smith.

Mrs. Fagon looked at me and then Dr. Smith. Mrs. Fagon knew Dr. Smith was my boss, and I could see in her eyes that she had something to say. I was sure Mrs. Fagon was going to tell Dr. Smith the truth about the delivery.

I cleared my throat and waited with anticipation. I saw my career flash before my eyes. At that moment, I knew how Dropsy felt every time someone teased him about the operating room. This was a golden moment for Mrs. Fagon, and I was sure she would shine. To my amazement, Mrs. Fagon turned to Nurse Iris and said calmly, "Nurse, may I please have something for pain? I need something. May I please have some pain medicine? Thank you, Nurse. I appreciate your kindness."

Nurse Iris and I both looked at Mrs. Fagon like she had three heads and was from the planet called Anywhere But Here. The Mrs. Fagon we had been dealing with was a cussing, fussing, and abusive son-of-a-gun. This Mrs. Fagon actually appeared civil.

Pain does strange things to people. Pain can change a person's entire personality. It turns some people from Mr. Hyde into Dr. Jekyll. Mrs. Fagon was a true example of the power of transformation. It was good to know that Mrs. Fagon could be polite and civilized. I was thankful for the sake of the new baby.

"Mrs. Fagon, I'll get you something for pain right away."

Nurse Iris was reading my mind. We definitely wanted to keep Mrs. Fagon quiet. At least until Dr. Smith walked out of the room. I did not want to take any chances of Mrs. Fagon transforming back into Dr. Jekyll and speaking what was really on her mind.

Dr. Smith was impressed, "Good job, Dr. Jones. You can give the group an update on breech deliveries in the Morning Report," She then left the room.

I let out a big sigh. Mrs. Fagon was a smoking gun, and I had just dodged a very lethal bullet. I got excited when I recalled Dr. Smith's compliment: "Good job Dr. Jones." However, the excitement was short-lived. My heart sank. My throat got dry. I turned to Nurse Iris and tried to speak. "Did ... Dr. Smith say she wanted me to present breech deliveries at the Morning Report?"

Nurse Iris smiled, "Yes she did. You can do it, Dr. Jones. Just remember the way you delivered this baby."

Mrs. Fagon started to laugh, "Ha, ha, ha! That doctor didn't know what she just *%#* did. I bet she can't even find her way out of an elevator in a two-story building. Ha, ha, ha! All she did was listen to the *%#* nurse give instructions. That doctor has no *%#* clue. Ha, ha, ha! That dumb trainee has no *%#* clue."

The Mrs. Fagon we knew was back. The sad part about it was that she was telling the truth. I didn't remember what I had just done.

"Iris, can you review the steps of breech delivery with me?"

I took out my note cards, planning to write down every word that Iris said. Nurse Iris said, "Remember."

Mrs. Fagon laughed so hard that she almost fell out of the bed. One thing was for certain: The pain medicine was working, and Mrs. Fagon was in no distress.

Mrs. Fagon continued, "She has no *%#* clue. That doctor has no *%#* clue how to deliver a butt-baby."

Mrs. Fagon laughed hysterically, "I just had a butt-baby, and that doctor has no *%#* clue how she did it. She has no clue how to deliver a butt-baby. I bet if she saw another butt-baby, she'd have a heart attack. She has no *%#* clue. Ha, ha, ha!"

Nurse Iris looked directly at me, "Dr. Jones, ignore Mrs. Fagon."

I looked at Medical Student Berney, even he began to laugh. Everyone in the room wanted to be a Saturday night comedian. I wanted to tell Berney a thing or two. How dare he make fun of me? Berney was a 325-pound wimp. He was scared of screaming mothers and yelling babies. I wanted to give Berney a piece of my mind. I wanted to tell him what I really thought about him and his sarcastic attitude. In my book, he was a loser. But, just as I was about to open my mouth, Nurse Iris interceded.

"The most important thing you need to remember about delivering a breech baby, is that you need to let the baby deliver on its own up to the (umbilicus belly button). If you pull too soon or too hard, the head or arm might get stuck. A safe breech delivery depends on the mother's pushing and your patience."[7]

"Thank you, Iris. I could not have done it without you."

"That's the truth. You have no *%#* clue on how to deliver a butt-baby. No clue I tell you. No *%#* clue. I hope I don't ever see your sorry self again."

Nurse Iris warned, "Dr. Jones, ignore Mrs. Fagon."

"Iris, thank you. Thank you very much."

"Next time you find yourself involved with a stressful delivery, take a deep breath, count to three, and tell yourself that you know what you're doing—even if you are the only one in the room to believe it."

"You got that right. She will be the only one in the room to believe that *%#* crap."

Nurse Iris continued, "Just act like you know what you're doing. You have to practice medicine using the 'Doctor's Mystique.'"

"Iris, what is the Doctor's Mystique?"

Mrs. Fagon couldn't resist, "Whatever it is, you definitely don't have it. You have no *%#* clue."

Medical Student Berney wanted to know, too: "What is the Doctor's Mystique?"

I looked at Berney and rolled my eyes. I gave him a look that told him exactly what was on my mind.

Nurse Iris answered, "Never let them see you sweat."

Mrs. Fagon shrieked with laughter, "I was right. Look at her over there shaking. She has no *%#* clue."

Mrs. Fagon began to cough from all the laughing.

"There was certainly no Doctor's Mystique during that particular delivery," I thought, "Sweat was dripping down my face, and my entire scrub top was soaking wet."

Nurse Iris continued, "Practice medicine without panic or sentimental value to the outcome."

"Nurse Iris, that sounds harsh."

"But it's not. That's how medicine works. The next breech delivery you encounter, you'll be able to coach someone else through it."

<u>See one</u>
<u>Do one</u>
<u>Teach one</u>

My problem was that this was my first breech delivery. I was seeing and doing at the same time. Now, Dr. Smith was expecting me to teach breech delivery techniques in the Morning Report. I was doomed.

My thoughts moved to the baby. That little baby had a really rough start, making his grand entrance into life. He was most certainly destined for greatness. Who knows, that little guy might grow up to be the president. One thing was for certain; he was definitely a fighter. That alone will take him far in life.

Mrs. Fagon asked, "Doc, what's your first name?"

I looked at Mrs. Fagon, "Are you talking to me?"

Mrs. Fagon replied, "You seem to be the only *%#* doctor in this room. Yes, I'm talking to you. What's your *%#* first name?"

I couldn't hold back any longer, "Mrs. Fagon, I am not using that language with you, so I would appreciate it if you kept your cussing and sarcastic comments to yourself. I don't want to hear them."

Mrs. Fagon replied "Ouch! Touchy…Touchy. You don't have to be so snappy. I didn't mean to offend you. I just want to know your first name."

I pointed to my name tag, "My name is Chandra."

Mrs. Fagon commented, "Strange name. What does it mean?"

I could not believe it. Mrs. Fagon was trying to be civil.

"Chandra is an Indian name. It means Moon Princess."

"Moon Princess my foot; I remember a dead girl named Chandra."

"I don't know what you are talking about, Mrs. Fagon."

"Nurse, you remember that dead girl?"

Nurse Iris continued to work and ignored Mrs. Fagon.

Mrs. Fagon pressed on, "Didn't they have a space shuttle that crashed named Chandra?"

"Not quite like that, Mrs. Fagon."

"Anyway, I like the name. I think I'll name my baby after you. This is number six, and I'm all out of family and friend names. Besides, I want to remember all this *%#* drama you put us through."

I shook my head in disbelief. I thought, "The drama I put you through? I believe it's the other way around." I could not believe my ears. Just five minutes ago Mrs. Fagon was yelling, cussing, and threatening to sue everybody in the delivery room. She had even claimed she would name the hospital Fagon South Central. But now she wanted to name her baby after me. Yeah... go figure!

Mrs. Fagon droned on. "I'll name him Shawn. Yeah, that sounds good. I will name him Shawn Ferdinane Fagon. Ferdinane is my maiden name, and it just flows. That's what we'll call him, little baby Shawn."

I didn't know whether to be flattered or frustrated.

"Dr. Jones, you know why she wants to name the baby after you?"

"No, Iris, I don't."

"This is her baby number six. She needs somebody to help with the bills and pay for college tuition. The next thing she'll do is ask you to be the baby's godparent."

"Really?"

"Yes, really. Don't get me wrong. It's a privilege to be a godparent, but I think it's a prerequisite to have some personal family ties."

I just laughed. That was the first time during the shift that I actually felt like laughing.

Then Mrs. Fagon sprung it on me: "Hey Doc, can I ask you something?"

"Yes, Mrs. Fagon."

"Since I'm naming my baby after you and all, will you be my baby's godmother?"

I looked at Nurse Iris.

Nurse Iris said, "I told you so. Some things never change. That's one of the oldest scams in the book. The patients love to get the new doctors fresh out of medical school. You've been a doctor all of two months. You're fresh bait."

"Mrs. Fagon, thank you for the honor, but I'm unable to be your baby's godmother."

Mrs. Fagon was quick to respond, "On second thought, Shawn Fagon does not sound so good. I really don't like that *%#* name."

She then looked at Medical Student Berney. "Hey you, Big Fella." Berney asked, "Who me?"

"Yes, you Big Fella. What's your first name?"

"My name is Berney."

"What's that mean?"

"I have no idea."

"I can think of a few choice meanings for his name," I thought, "'Useless' and 'Shifty' come to mind."

"Here we go again. Mrs. Fagon, leave the medical student alone. He's not going to be your baby's god-anything. Just name the kid Fredrick. Fredrick goes with Fagon, and it means Ruler. Name him Fredrick Fagon."

"Fredrick—Ruler. I like that. His name will be Fredrick Fagon."

We walked out of the delivery room.

"Iris, how did you come up with the name Fredrick and Ruler?"

"The patient in the other room named her son Fredrick. I overheard her say that the name was German for Ruler."

We both laughed. After what that little boy went through, he definitely deserved the name *Ruler*. I wonder whatever happened to Fredrick Fagon. Who knows, Fredrick might become the next president. I think of great men of valor… if not the president, then possibly the next Bill Gates, Dr. Henry Foster, or Bishop TD Jakes.

I sometimes think of Mrs. Fagon's threats. She wanted to name the hospital Fagon South Central and put all the staff on welfare. It has been over 25 years since that dramatic experience and Fredrick Fagon must be doing well. I still have plenty to eat, and the hospital is still standing. I laugh. "What am I thinking? That was just an everyday occurrence at the General."

Chapter 4

My Father

It has been two months since my meeting with Dr. Beta, and I have spent the majority of my time in bed. The beta blockers are kicking my butt. My energy is gone, and all I do is sleep. Private practice has become too stressful. I quit my job, and now I am trying to rebuild my life. I get sad when I think about my dad, now that I am sharing his fate. I am transported back in time and see the vision so clearly.

My father, Sergeant Calvin Jones, always looked so proud in his United States Military uniform. My dad looked so handsome in his official dress blue attire.

I am taken back to Thanksgiving morning. Thanksgiving was my family's favorite holiday. On one particular year, I was planning a trip to Jamaica with Charmaine Clark, my friend and colleague. I waited so late to buy my plane ticket that by the time I attempted to make my reservations, the price was out of my budget.

That Thanksgiving morning I walked into the kitchen. My mother greeted me with a big hug and a kiss.

"Chandra, please go and wake up your father. Breakfast will be ready in about ten minutes."

I looked at the clock. It was 10:00 a.m.

"Looks like Dad and I both overslept."

"You both were tired, so I let you sleep. Now go and wake up your father and tell him to get up for breakfast."

I walked out of the kitchen, down the hallway, and into my parents' bedroom. As I entered the room, a cold chill hit me. I looked around. At first glance, I didn't see my father. The television set was on, and the volume was so loud that it hurt my ears. I slowly walked around the side of the bed, which was facing the door.

As I turned the corner, I looked down and saw my father on the floor. He was lying face down and was wedged between the nightstand and the bed. I tried to move him, but it was a struggle. Although my dad weighed 180 pounds and was 5' 10", he felt like he weighed a ton. He was stiff, and his body felt cold. I gave it all I had, and I managed to pull him away from the nightstand. I then turned him over and laid him on his back. I went immediately into doctor mode and started to perform CPR (Cardiac Pulmonary Resuscitation).[8,9]

My mind began to spin out of control. A million thoughts bombarded me at the same time. What happened to my father? Why didn't I hear him fall? I was in the room next door. When did he fall? What happened? How did this happen?

I told myself to snap out of it. I had to help my dad. My medical training took over, and I reminded myself of the drill:

ABC-ABC-ABC

A: Airway = Check the airway
B: Breathing = Check for breathing
C: Circulation = Check for pulse

I knelt down next to my father and began to shake his shoulder. I prayed he would hear me and open his eyes.

"Dad! Dad! Can you hear me? Dad, wake up! Dad, can you hear me? Dad, please wake up! Dad please, please, wake up!"

My mother entered the room and started to scream. She was hysterical and I couldn't concentrate on my father and her at the same time. I looked into my mother's eyes. I struggled to find the words to tell her to call 911.

Mother asked, "What happened? What happened?"

I could no longer control myself and began to cry.

"Mom, call 911! Dad needs help! Call 911 now!"

My mother left the room. I heard her go down the hall, crying hysterically.

I turned my attention back to my father. I opened his mouth. The airway was clear. I next checked for breathing. I remember the pneumonic: <u>Look, Listen, Feel.</u> I put my ear to my father's face. I couldn't hear him breathing. I couldn't feel him breathing. I looked at his chest. I strained desperately to see movement, but there was none.

I tilted my father's head back and lifted his chin. Time was now moving in slow motion. I filled up my lungs with as much air as I could. I gave my father two quick breaths, hoping that the life in me would help my dad. I had to believe it would. I couldn't give up.

I looked at his chest. No movement. No movement. My father's body was still. I placed my hand on my father's neck to check for a pulse. His neck was cold. There was no pulse. I felt nothing. I positioned my hands in the center of his chest. My arms were shaking. My hands were numb. I didn't care. I wouldn't give up. I couldn't give up.

I pushed down on his chest and begin the count. 1 and 2 and 3 and... and 15. I continued with two breaths and fifteen chest compressions. My mind began to play tricks on me. Is it two breaths and fifteen chest compressions, or is it two breaths and thirty chest compressions?

I was reminded of Dr. Cyril Moore in medical school. He would always say, "**In medicine, make things make sense**."

How long could I hold my breath without breathing? Not very long. Two breaths with fifteen chest compressions made sense to me. I continued with two and fifteen. I started the count: 1 and 2 and 3 and… and 15. I was on round ten when the paramedics walked into the room. My arms were throbbing, and my hands were blue. I didn't care. All I could think about was saving my dad's life. I couldn't give up. I had to do my best.

I looked up and saw Shaw Williams in his paramedic uniform. Shaw and I both graduated from the same high school. Shaw became a paramedic when he got out of the military. I was so happy to see him. I tried to muster a smile, but my mouth wouldn't cooperate. My eyes showed my pain, and my face revealed my sorrow.

Shaw explained, "We just got the call. We came as fast as we could. Chandra, what happened to your father?"

Trying hard to fight back the tears, I struggled to say, "I just found him on the floor this morning. I don't know what happened. I walked into the room to wake him up for breakfast, and I found him on the floor. I don't know how long he's been lying here. I just walked into the room to wake him up for breakfast." My hands were trembling, and my voice continued to crack.

"Shaw, I tried CPR, and it's not working. Shaw, it's not working. Please help. Please help us."

Shaw grabbed me by the shoulder. "Chandra, let me take over. It'll be okay."

"But, but, but—he's not breathing. Shaw, I tried, but he's not breathing."

I moved out of the way as Shaw knelt down beside my father. He touched his neck to check for a pulse. I could see in Shaw's eyes that the life in my father was gone. The eyes never lie.

Shaw called to his partner, "Craig, I need you to get the oxygen and the defibrillator from the truck." Craig left the room and walked out to the truck. People were starting to gather in the house. I could hear my mother screaming. I could tell there was a crowd in the living room.

Shaw attempted to take my mind off what we both knew was obvious.

"Does your father have any medical problems?"

My voice was barely a whisper, "My father has high blood pressure but no other medical problems."

"What medication is your father taking?"

"I don't know? I'll have to ask my mother."

"Does your father have any allergies?"

I looked into Shaw's eyes. My tears continued to fall. I knew the questions were routine. We both knew it was too late for a history of medical problems, medications, or allergies.

The eyes were silent, yet they spoke volumes of comprehensible words. I could read Shaw's eyes loud and clear.

Craig walked back into the room carrying the oxygen and the defibrillator. Craig hooked up the oxygen mask and then placed the mask over my father's face. At the same time, Shaw attached the chest leads. He then looked at me. I saw the painful truth in his eyes. We both knew what would happen when the machine was turned on.

I took a deep breath. My heart stood still. I looked for hope. I looked for a gesture. I looked for a sign. My vision was cloudy. I wiped the tears away from my eyes so I could see. I looked, and then I listened. The screen showed a dot. One green dot in a sea of black. I held my breath. I wiped my eyes. The signal appeared and it was flat. I told myself my eyes were deceiving me. My ears wouldn't lie. I listened with all my strength. There was no sound. Shaw saw my despair and turned up the volume on the monitor. We both listened.

Beeeeeeeeeeeeeeeeep

Dr. T would always say, "In medicine the inevitable will become obvious." She was right. I looked at the machine. I looked at my dad's face. All signs of life were gone. He was really gone. I just broke down. My fear was real...

"Shaw it can't be. This can't be happening."

Shaw grabbed me. I buried my head into his shoulder and continued to cry.

"I'm sorry, I wish there was something we could do. I'm so sorry."

After what seemed like an eternity, Shaw and Craig left the room. My mother entered the bedroom, and we just held each other.

When I reflect on that dreadful day even now, I still can't believe it. It is almost like it was yesterday. My dad was only fifty-seven years old. My dad had been diagnosed with high blood pressure, and he died with an enlarged heart. It appears my heart condition is congenital. This morning my pressure is okay. At least the medicine is working.

I take a deep breath, look in the mirror, and wipe the tears from my eyes. I was daddy's girl, and I still can't believe he is gone.

Chapter 5

Back to Work

F ive months later.
   It had been a long night, and I could not sleep.

My body requires eight hours of sleep for maximum efficiency. My body requires six hours of sleep for adequate performance. Most days, I have to settle for four hours of sleep. Last night was a four-hour-sleep night. It was going to be a long day.

Mr. Alarm Clock: beep, beep—Louder—Beep—Louder—BEEP, BEEP

The sound from my particular alarm clock sends shock waves through the entire room. Those last few minutes of sleep are precious, and I try desperately to savor them. My problem is simple. I have never, and probably never will, win the war for more sleep.

I look at the clock: 5:00 a.m.

I smack the snooze button, close my eyes, and immediately fall right back to sleep.

Mr. Alarm Clock: beep, beep—Louder—Beep—Louder—BEEP, BEEP BEEPBEEPBEEP!

I reach blindly for the snooze button and *thump!* The clock falls off the night stand and hits the floor. Silence. Good. I pull the blanket over my head and fall back to sleep.

Pound!—Pound!—Pound!—Pound!

My ten-minute wish disappears when I hear my mother's fist beating on the door like a drum. She is either going to bruise her fist or tear down my door. Either way, I'm sure the people around the corner can hear the pounding.

Pound! Pound! POUND! POUND!

Next I hear my mother's voice, "Chandra, time to start moving."

Some people always wake up happy. Me, I'm just happy to wake up.

Pound! Pound! Pound! POUND! POUND! POUND!

The bedroom door opens, and a strobe that bears resemblance to a police search-and-rescue floodlight burns my eyes. I squint, and my head begins to throb immediately.

Some people have no sympathy. Some people have no mercy. Some people—A train clangs loudly along the nearby railroad tracks.

Tooooooot! Tooooooot! Tooooooot! Tooooooot!

This morning, it seems I am not to catch a break. The clock tortures my ears, the spotlight blinds me, and that train is harassment, plain and simple.

"Chandra, get up," Mother calls out. "You don't want to be late for your appointment with Dr. Von."

Dr. Von, Chairman of OB/GYN at Mercy General Hospital, called me just last night: "Hello, may I speak to Dr. Jones?"

"Dr. Von, is that you? It's good to hear your voice."

Dr. Von is my mentor, second mother, and the reason I am in Maternal Fetal Medicine.

Dr. Von said, "I heard you left the private practice group. Those guys have no morals. They have no respect in the academic medical community. There's a rumor they're being investigated by the feds. It's a good thing you got out."

"Thanks."

"What are you doing with yourself these days?" "I've been trying to study for my oral boards." "What about work?"

"I've been home for five months."

Dr. Von's voice was firm. "Time for you to get back to work. I need some help here at the General. I want you to come back and run the Transport Service on Labor and Delivery."

"I'm not sure I'm ready. I'll try to help until you find someone permanent, but I can only work part-time. I can't work those long shifts anymore."

"That can be arranged. I need for you to start right away. Come to my office tomorrow morning at 7:00 a.m., and we can set up your schedule."

That was all great last night, but today, my big return to medicine has not begun well. I cover my face with the pillow. It's a hopeless attempt, but I try desperately to shield my eyes from the supernova blazing in the hallway. The door opens wider, and the brightness in my room intensifies. The light is so bright that all of the shadows scream and run for cover.

What a way to start the morning; or, should I say, what a way *not* to start the morning. With all this drama, I really don't want to wake up, get out of the bed, or talk to Dr. Von. I sit up in the bed and look around.

"Mom, I'm up, I'm moving."

I say to myself, "I'll get up in ten. I need ten more minutes of snoozing."

Mother answers, "Breakfast will be ready soon. I'll call you when it's on the table."

The door closes, and the spotlight is gone. The sound from the train has finally disappeared, and the stillness returns. I fall back in the bed and once again pull the covers over my head. My thoughts drift to my Grandmother's wisdom. Her voice has a way of popping in my head when I feel stressed: "Life has a way of tenderizing the tough." Grandmother was certainly right. Life has a way of turning things around—tenderizing the tough. Everything in my life is now different.

<u>Mr. Alarm Clock</u>

Beep, Beep (Louder) Beep (Louder) Beep, Beep!

I pick the alarm clock up from the floor and reach for my medication. I take a big gulp of water and sigh deeply.

Why is this happening? Just last year, I thought life was perfect. I was planning a wedding, starting a new medical practice, and enjoying perfect health. I was so happy, but suddenly things fell apart. My engagement ended in something that resembled a scene from Tyler Perry's movie *Diary of an Angry Black Woman,* my venture in private practice blew up in my face, my cardiologist has me on heart medication and, to top it all off, I am going back to the General.

I turn on my bedside lamp and reach for my *Life Application Study Bible* that I always leave on the bed next to me. I read the Proverb for the day. Today is January 10.

> The godly are showered with blessings;
> The words of the wicked conceal violent intentions.
> (Proverbs 10:6)[5]

I say to myself, "After all I have been through, I need this reassurance. Maybe things are finally starting to look up. Maybe going back to the General is just what I need."

I grab my wrist blood pressure cuff to take my pressure.

Beep—110/70 (Optimal blood pressure < 120/80).

I'm starting out this morning okay. At least the medication is working. I crawl out of bed and rub the last hope of sleep out of my eyes. I grab the remote control for the TV and turn it on. I look for the weather station and flip through several channels. The temperature in January can be very unpredictable. I continue to flip through the channels. My forehead wrinkles and my eyes open wide when I see the words:

Special News Bulletin

The news anchor is standing in front of the General. I think I am seeing things… not Mercy General. I stare at the news anchor, but I can't put a name to his face. I believe I know him from somewhere, but I just can't remember. I turn up the volume on the TV and listen.

"This is a special report. It is now confirmed that the doctors at Mercy General Hospital are planning to leave the hospital at 8:00 a.m. this morning. I repeat, the doctors at Mercy

General Hospital are planning to leave the hospital at 8:00 a.m. this morning. Stay tuned to Channel 12 News."

I change the station…no luck. I can't find out any more information about what is happening at the General. I think to myself, "No one life can have this much drama. What is this really about?"

I walk into the bathroom and turn on the shower. Even the hot water can't revive me. My eyes slowly open. The water feels so good on my aching neck and back. The steam begins to bring relief to my pounding head. My sinuses slowly begin to open. Now I can breathe. I inhale the vapors. I exhale the stress. As the water hits my body, it begins to vitalize my senses. I am finally beginning to wake up. This is good. The tension is starting to lift.

I emerge from the comfort of the shower and sit on the vanity stool facing the mirror. I can't get the vision of the General out of my mind. I can't get the words *Special News Bulletin* out of my head. I can't get the concept of a strike out of my thoughts.

I look at the mirror with a blank stare of confusion. I say to myself, "Mirror, Mirror talk to me. Mirror, Mirror talk to me."

A few minutes of wishful thinking soon fade away. My hopes of this being a bad dream are shattered and disappear. I say to the mirror, "Mirror, if you did speak I'd probably think I was staring in the face of a crazy woman… Silence, good. At least I can say with certainty that I am not crazy. With all this drama, I can at least count on my sanity."

The mirror begins to cast a spell on me. I'm now paralyzed in time. I'm frozen in the moment. I can't move; I can't breathe; I can't see. I feel as though my mind is starting to play tricks on me. As I stare deeper into the mirror a vision of the General appears.

Chapter 6

Mercy General Hospital

I see the frightening face of Resident Priscilla Coleman. Priscilla was a year ahead of me at medical school. For some reason, Priscilla, Medical Student Berney, Nurse Iris, and I always got stuck working together. Priscilla treated all the interns like dog waste. Some days we got treated worse than crap. Priscilla's strategy was simple: she was miserable and irritated everybody. Working with Priscilla was dangerous. Around Priscilla the truth always changed.

I remember an occasion when a patient had come into the triage area with her cervix dilated to 10 centimeters. I examined the patient and could not tell if the head, butt, leg, or arm was coming first. It's vital that you know the position of the baby when attempting delivery because this will determine if the baby will be delivered safely from below (vaginal) or if the baby has to be delivered from above (abdomen via C-section). One way to check the position of the baby is to use Leopold's Maneuvers to assess the mother. I opened my book and looked up Leopold's Maneuvers. Medical Student Berney entered the room.

"Dr. Jones, what is going on?" He asked.

"I need to determine the baby's position. I want you to read the instructions for me," I handed Berney the book.

"Leopold number 1: palpate the top of the uterus (fundus) and check to see what is presenting."

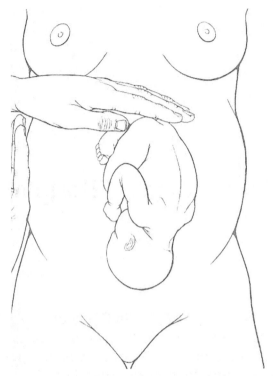

Leopold Maneuver #1 (Source: *Obstetrics—Normal and Problem Pregnancies, 4th Edition*, 2002, 367).[7]

I placed my hands on the top of the uterus. The patient's belly was so large, I didn't know what I was feeling. I tried really hard, but it was useless.

The patient looked on in disbelief. "Oh, hell no! I am having a baby and I don't want two trainees in the room!"

Reassuringly, Nurse Iris told her, "Calm down. The doctor knows what she's doing."

"If she does, why is the medical student reading from a book?"

All eyes turned to Berney. With a lump in my throat and a squeak to my voice, I struggled to say, "Berney, read step number 2."

"Leopold number 2: palpate the sides of the maternal abdomen. Feel for the fetal spine and the small parts (arms and legs).

"Step number 2! Oh, hell no... I said get me a real doctor!"

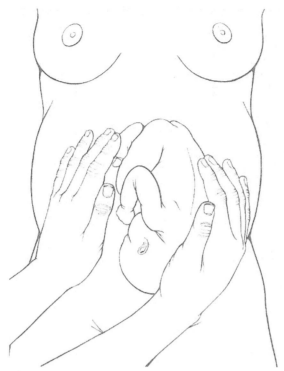

Leopold Maneuver # 2 (Source: *ObstetricsNormal and Problem Pregnancies*, 4th Edition, 2002, 367).[7]

This did not go any better. I couldn't find the small parts. There was too much space between the uterus and skin.

"Okay, Berney, read step 3."

"Leopold number 3: place fingers above the maternal pubic bone (symphysis pubis) and top of the uterus (fundus). The fetal breech is often larger, softer, and more palpable than the fetal head."

I followed the instructions. There was no way I could tell the difference between the butt and the head. It was hopeless.

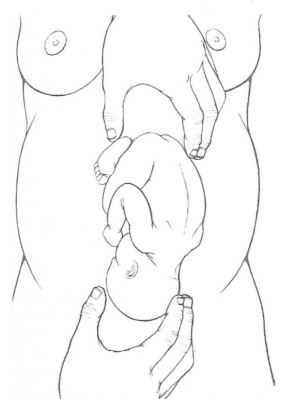

Leopold Maneuver # 3 (Source: *Obstetrics—Normal and Problem Pregnancies, 4th Edition*, 2002, 367).[7]

"Berney, what is the next step?"

"Leopold number 4: face the patient and move the hands along the pubic bone (anterior superior iliac crest) to determine the presentation of the fetus."

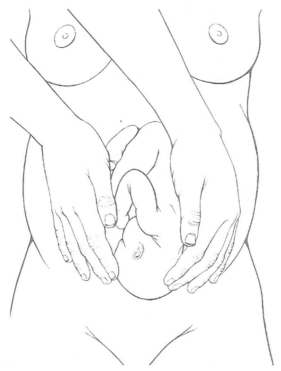

Leopold Maneuver number 4 (Source: *Obstetrics—Normal and Problem Pregnancies, 4th Edition*, 2002, 367).[7]

I could not feel the baby. I knew the baby was in there somewhere, but my hands could not find the little one. I had no clue what position the baby was in by palpating the abdomen. The only way to tell the fetal position for certain was to view the fetus using the ultrasound machine. I had to know the fetal position to determine the delivery route. In this case, a picture would be worth a thousand words.

"Berney, I need you to go and get the ultrasound machine."

Berney returned with the ultrasound.

I performed a quick scan to check the fetal position. I looked at the screen. The head was at the top and the butt was at the bottom. The baby was breech. My suspicions were right. This was the patient's first baby. It was too risky to deliver the baby from below. The plan was to cut, and it was time for some real action.

I reported my findings to Resident Priscilla Coleman and waited in anticipation for her to call surgery. I just knew, since this was the patient's first baby, and the patient's first surgery, Priscilla would let me do some cutting. I am a surgeon and a surgeon in training always wants to cut. I was ready…finally some real action on Labor and Delivery. I was eager to put my fingers on the blade and show off my one-handed surgical knot skills.

To everyone's horror, Priscilla called the Attending Physician and said that the patient's cervix was completely dilated and that the baby was delivering head first. I thought I was hearing things. I was confused. I once again told Priscilla that the position of the baby was breech. Priscilla Coleman just ignored me. She did not even acknowledge that I was talking to her. I knew the baby was breech. Berney knew the baby was breech. Nurse Iris knew the baby was breech. The patient even knew the baby was breech. We had all seen the position of the baby on the ultrasound machine... or at least I thought we had all seen the same thing.

I said to Priscilla once again, "The baby is breech. Did you hear me? I said the patient is breech."

"Jones, I examined the baby and my examination is the only one that counts."

I reminded myself, "Priscilla is the boss. She has more experience than me. I guess she knows what she is doing."

When the Attending Physician arrived, Priscilla again told him that the patient was delivering head first.

The delivery was an obstetrical nightmare. We rolled the patient to the delivery room and placed her legs up in the stirrups. She started to push, and the water bag with the amniotic fluid around the baby broke as soon as she did so. The amniotic fluid missed the drapes and flew everywhere. I got completely soaked. Thank goodness for the face shield and delivery boots.

The Attending asked the nurse to check the fetal heart tones. Nurse Iris placed the monitor on the abdomen. She was unable to pick up the baby's heartbeat. Talk about scary. Everyone in the delivery room held their breath.

No heart tones.

The Attending asked me to examine the patient.

I examined the patient, and I felt a hand full of the baby's umbilical cord. Yes, cord prolapse.

Cord Prolapse is a true obstetrical emergency—or should I say a true obstetrical *nightmare*. The fetal umbilical cord is the baby's lifeline. The cord carries the oxygenated blood to the baby from the mother, and the umbilical cord also returns the blood that is used by the baby back to the mother. It functions like a recycling interstate highway.

When the umbilical cord delivers before the baby, the oxygen to the baby can be cut off. The baby requires constant blood flow to stay alive. A mother can carry a fetus for nine months and be perfectly healthy, but during the delivery a cord prolapse can cause a baby to lose its life or suffer the consequences of severe brain damage within a matter of minutes.

All doctors learn to respect the words *cord prolapse*. A cord prolapse will send chills through the spine of the most skilled doctor. Yes, a cord prolapse is an obstetrical nightmare. When I announced cord prolapse, everyone started to move. No questions were asked. Everyone in the room knew the dreaded consequences of not delivering this baby within a matter of minutes.

The anesthesiologist immediately put the patient to sleep. My job was to keep my hand in the birth canal to protect the umbilical cord from compression. It was my job to make sure that the blood was still flowing adequately through the umbilical cord. I was scared, but I was determined to protect this baby's life. The life of this baby was literally in my hands.

One minute after the patient was put to sleep, the Attending pulled the baby out of the abdomen. I was under the drapes holding the umbilical cord. All I could hear was slash, slash, and the baby was out. The Attending cut the baby out so fast, he almost cut my hand. I am sure that I let go of the umbilical cord just as the knife was nearing my fingers.

I remember the words of the Attending, "Dr. Jones you can come out from under the surgical drapes now. The baby has been delivered."

I looked around the room. I saw the baby under the warmer. The baby had survived. Yes, the baby had survived. That day I saw the power of a miracle before my very eyes. The baby survived and experienced no complications from the cord prolapse.

With today's legal system, vaginal breech deliveries are few and far between for young doctors in training. The old saying is that people don't sue for a life undamaged echoes from doctor in training to doctor in training. These days, the only doctors who are skilled in performing vaginal breech deliveries are the pioneers of yesterday. The doctors in training today just don't have the patient population to be trained proficiently. Vaginal breech deliveries are just too risky. With law suits at an all-time high, doctors practice defensive medicine. Some people call it medicine with a conscience. I prefer to call it practicing medicine as a patient advocate.

Priscilla was true to form. Following the delivery, she told the Attending Physician that I was to blame for not knowing the presentation of the baby. When she realized that no one in the room believed her story, she changed it. She claimed the baby flipped around before the surgery. It was obvious to everyone in the room that Priscilla was lying. Priscilla knew the patient was breech. Nurse Iris, Berney, and I knew the patient was breech. The fly on the wall knew the baby was breech. All Priscilla cared about was the breech extraction. Yes, at the expense of the patient and the baby, Priscilla wanted to practice delivering a vaginal breech baby before she got into the real world.

Nurse Iris informed the Attending Physician of the ultrasound examination and the findings of the breech baby. After being caught, Priscilla finally confessed to the Attending. That day, Priscilla had to face up to the music, and she declared all-out war on me.

Yes, around Priscilla Coleman the truth has a way of changing. Working with Priscilla I learned the art of covering my back. In medicine, this art has served me well. Not only do I cover my back, but I cover my side, front, face, and especially my throat. People have a way of always trying to go for the jugular, the large blood vessel at the side of your neck that gives oxygen to your brain.

Chapter 7

Morning Breakfast

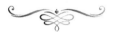

The spell is broken when I hear my mother's voice: "Chandra, breakfast is on the table. Come and eat before everything gets cold."

I can feel the weight and stress of the moment beginning to lift. I look in the mirror one last time and say to myself, "I am going to the General to talk to Dr. Von about part-time work. I will help out until she can find someone permanent. I owe her that much. I am only doing this out of my great admiration, respect, and loyalty to her. What is the harm in working one week each month—or, at the most, two?"

I wash my face with cold water and quickly apply my make-up: eyeliner, eyeshadow, and clear lip gloss—quick and easy. I comb my hair and tie it into a ponytail. I spruce up my school-girl image by sculpturing a few curls across my face. I don't make a big fuss with my hair. My style is simple: pulled back and functional. When I want to look fancy, I dress up my hair with a pretty clip-on bow. Today I'll wear the red one. Red is my color. It helps to add spice to my exciting life. We all can use a little more spice. It keeps things interesting.

I am once again reminded of my Grandmother's wisdom: "Dress like a million bucks and keep smiling. A smile will keep your associates *wondering* and your adversaries *clueless*."

As I look into the mirror, I say to myself: "I definitely look the part."

I smile. The tears are starting to fade. It is a good feeling. I am now awake and completely functional.

Today, I am wearing my black-and-white designer suit from the Dr. Jones Original Designs collection. For special effects, I will adorn the suit with a red sweater and black with white stripe scarf. I look down at my feet. Although the black pumps are made by Easy Spirit, I know that they will make walking up and down the halls of Mercy General

Hospital problematic. Those pumps will be murder on my feet. I don't want those swollen intern legs back. In my line of business as an obstetrician, that is a definite guarantee.

I could never understand how Dr. Tennison wore her pretty designer high heel shoes and pearl necklace in the operating room. She was definitely an operating room fashion icon. I walk in the closet and pick up my bright red clogs. Yes, I need to take my old trusty walking shoes. I put on my pearl necklace with matching earrings and smile as I remind myself, "If I take care of my feet, then I just know that my feet will take care of me."

I collect the remainder of my things and walk down the stairs. As I enter the kitchen, I smell pancakes from the griddle.

"Mom, it smells good. Strawberries and pancakes are my favorite. Thanks."

I sit at the table.

"Did you see the news this morning? I only caught a quick glimpse. Appears to be some problem at the General. Turn the TV to Channel 12 to see if the story is back on."

Mother said, "Something strange is always going on at that place. They say…"

"Mom, I am going there today to talk to Dr. Von, remember?"

"Yes, dear, I am sorry. Better turn on the TV to see what is happening."

Mother walks over to the television set and turns the station to Channel 12. The view of the General is in the background, and the camera is focused on the news anchor.

"Mom, that news anchor looks very familiar, but I can't place him."

"That is Charles Storey. He is the new anchor for Channel 12 News. He came back to town six months ago. I remember you and his younger brother, Tim, went to school together."

"That's his name, Charles Storey. This morning when I saw his face, I thought he looked familiar, but I couldn't remember where I knew him from."

"I wonder what happened to Tim. He was such a charming young fellow. I remember Tim had a paper route, sold greens from his mother's garden, collected the numbers for his father, and ripped off the old ladies in the community by taking their money for running errands. That boy was enterprising, a born hustler and miniature gangster con artist. I'm sure he went far in life; that is, if he stayed out of the penitentiary."

"Mom, I don't know what happened to Tim. We were schoolmates a long time ago. I haven't really kept up with any of my old high school friends. I've been so busy with medicine. Now that I'm back in town, I hope to see some of my old buddies."

"Mrs. Baker's daughter, Phoebe, works at the funeral home. Every family in this neighborhood has buried somebody at May's Mortuary within the last two years. Check with Phoebe, if Tim is still around, she can find him."

"Good idea. I'll get in touch with Phoebe. I would love to see her. Speaking of Tim, I am sure he's happily married with a lot of kids."

"And if he's not?"

"Mom it's time to change the subject. All I want to think about is what is happening at the General."

My mother looks up and points to the television screen. "There he is, Charles Storey is back on the screen. Charles really looks good. The whole community is so happy he's back in town."

I see my mother smile with the same pride that is usually reserved for bragging about family members. She continues, "The last news anchor on Channel 12 News had a terrible problem speaking. It was a mixture of stuttering with a speech impediment. It was something to hear. I stopped watching Channel 12 News, because I couldn't understand what the man was saying. I don't mean to talk about anyone's shortcomings because, Lord knows, we all have them. But I tell you one thing: He would probably still have his job if he was holding the camera and not talking to it. Talking to the camera cost that poor man his job, and Channel 12 News lost a lot of their viewers. With Charles on the tube, I bet the ratings are much better. If nothing else, he looks and sounds better."

We both look at the small television screen.

"Mom, turn up the volume. I want to hear what Charles is saying."

My mother pulls out the pliers from the cabinet. She grabs the broken knob on the television set and struggles to turn up the volume. On top of the television is a wire hanger. The antenna has been missing for the last two years.

"Mom, when are you going to get a new television set?"

"I am not in the kitchen long enough to watch television. This TV works fine. The knob is broken, and the antenna fell off, but the picture still looks good on three stations. Besides, if it worries you so much, why don't you buy me a new one? I want a new, forty-two-inch plasma flatscreen TV, one of those new fancy digital ones."

My mother pulls out a sales flier from the cabinet drawer and points to one of the pictures on the advertising page. "This one is nice, and it is a good bargain. The bargain is so good; you get two TVs for the price of one of those really big large screens. It sure would be nice to have a new TV in the kitchen and one in my bedroom. You know I am starting to have problems with my eyes, the doctor said."

Now she is really playing hardball. We both know that the doctor didn't say anything about me buying my mother a big-screen television set. I look at my mother.

"Don't start telling stories on your doctor. This is the New Year. Be good."

"The doctor did not exactly say I need a big-screen TV, but he did say to avoid eye strain."

"That is what they are calling it these days? Eye strain?"

The entire conversation is comical, and I begin to laugh.

My mother ignores me and continues with her motherly logic. "Let me know when you want to go shopping. The mall has great sales, and I'm available this weekend from noon until 5:00 p.m. I have a hair appointment and need to run some errands. This week is Reverend Johnson's anniversary, and I want to look really nice. I think the Pastor's Aide committee is planning to wear white. I need a new white suit."

She holds out her hand, "Can you advance me the cash?"

My mother is definitely on a fishing expedition now. First two new television sets and now a new suit. If I stick around here long enough, I just know that she'll hit me up for her hair appointment.

"Oh, by the way. I have a new stylist and…"

"Okay, Mom, I got the message."

"Today at 5:00 p.m. I plan to meet Ella at bingo. Tonight is the Big Game Special for $50,000. I want to get there early and get a good seat, so I can see the board. Sitting up front helps ease my eye strain."

I say to myself, "Here we go again with the eye strain story. My mother is milking this for all it is worth."

Mother holds out her hand, "Looks like Christmas and my December birthday have come again. I can't wait to tell Penny, Ella, and Viola about my new theater room with all the bells and whistles."

I interrupt my mother's train of thought and ask, "Do you know what's happening at the General?"

"That place stays in and out of the news. Something strange is always happening there."

"Like what?"

"There has been talk around town that the doctors are planning a strike."

"Really?"

"I've heard different stories. Mrs. Marshall at the grocery store told me all the doctors were going on strike. Mrs. Kennedy at the beauty salon told me it was just the baby doctors going on strike. Mrs. Ella at the bingo hall told me it was only the nurses going on strike. Mrs. Mays said …"

I interrupt, "Okay, Mom, I got the picture. It doesn't sound like any of your friends have the full story. It sounds like a lot of confused gossip."

"Make fun of my friends all you want. I told you I didn't know, but I do know one thing: Doctors walking out on their patients is not right. People abandoning their responsibilities is just plain wrong. What happened to the Oath of Hypocrites you pledged in med school?"

"It is the Hippocratic Oath, not the Oath of Hypocrites. Mom, if I didn't know you better, I would swear you're being sarcastic."

"If the doctors walk out of Mercy General, it may as well be the Oath of Hypocrites. If you ask me, doctors leaving patients and abandoning their responsibilities are hypocrites, and if you leave your patients, then that makes you a hypocrite, too. Nothing good will come of it—absolutely nothing. They are all Hippocratic Hypocrites."

I start to laugh. "Hippocratic Hypocrites? Only you, Mom, would think of that one."

"Yes, Hippocratic Hypocrites. That's what they are."

My attention turns to the events of the upcoming day. "I still can't believe all this is happening at Mercy General. What makes all this worse, is that Dr. Von did not mention the possibility of a strike yesterday."

I remember my grandmother's wisdom: "Evil comes in the form of a conspiracy or ambush." Is this what she meant? If nothing else, I definitely feel like I've been ambushed.

"Chandra, if someone said the doctors were planning a strike, would you be willing to help Dr. Von at the General?"

"You have a point."

"You talked about one administrator so bad, that I swore she walked around with a pitch fork in her hands. I just knew that poor lady had horns sticking out of the side of her neck. If you were told of the fire, would you seriously want to walk into the flames?"

I shake my head.

"I know you're concerned. Just go and talk to Dr. Von before you draw any conclusions. She's your mentor. She'll tell you the truth."

"Mom, you are right. I need to wait and speak to Dr. Von."

We both stare at the news.

Charles appears, "This is Charles Storey reporting live from Mercy General Hospital located on Mercy Boulevard in the commerce district. I am told that today is the last day to reach a compromise regarding the Family Center Care Policy. The OB/GYN physicians are still threatening to leave the hospital at 8:00 a.m. today if their demands are not met. I understand there will be one last meeting this morning with the administrators and the OB/GYN staff. We are informed that if a compromise is not reached, it will not be good news for Mercy General Hospital. At the present time we are unable to reach any of the administrators or any of the physicians involved in the strike. Both sides appear to be cloaked in silence. We can only hope for the best."

Mother and I both stare intently at the television screen.

"This is Charles Storey with Channel 12 News… wait a minute, here comes one of the administrators now." Charles then directs Barry, the camera man, to focus on Mr. Tight-Check, the Chief Financial Officer of Mercy General Hospital. Mr. Tight-Check holds up his briefcase to avoid the camera.

"Mr. Tight-Check can you give us a statement? Can you tell the viewers the latest update on the Family Center Care Policy?"

"I have no comment. Leave me alone. Turn off that camera, and get off our property. If you don't leave, I'll call the police." Mr. Tight-Check swings his briefcase at Barry. The screen goes blank.

"Mom, did you see that administrator swing at the camera man on live TV? It looks like things are really out of control."

"Yes it does, and Charles is on top of the story. At least we can hear what he is saying. That last news anchor…"

"Mom, you said you were going to be nice."

"You're right. I have some news from a more reliable source. You know Mrs. Jacobs at the pharmacy? Her sister told Molly that Sonya said Charles and his wife are expecting their first baby. You would be great as the baby's doctor."

"Mom, I am not a pediatrician, and I really hope they don't need the help of a high-risk obstetrician. If, for some reason, they do need my services, I'll be sure to tell them that you referred me to them."

"You got a deal, and I expect my referral fee in cash. As a matter of fact, I will take my advance now."

"Mom I need to get going. I don't want to be late for my meeting with Dr. Von."

As I walk away from the table, a cold chill hits me. I turn and look at my mother.

"Chandra I am glad you are home. I know things have been rough for you, and now you are walking into a hornet's nest."

The harsh reality hits me. This nightmare is real. If I didn't feel bad before, after hearing this line-up of problems, I can be sure of one thing: I qualify for the home for special people and the insanity plea could be used if I go postal.

I walk over to my mother, and we give each other a strong embrace. Tears fill my eyes as I remember how close I came to losing my mother, best friend, and precious jewel.

Chapter 8

Memories of Mother

I flinch as I remember the image of my mother lying in the bed in the Cardiac Intensive Care Unit. It was the day of my OB/GYN residency graduation. My mother had flown into town three days before the ceremony.

Mrs. Hattie Shinult, my surrogate mother and Director of Labor and Delivery, was kind enough to invite my mother to stay at her home while she was in town. Hattie knew that I lived in the nursing dormitory across the street from the hospital and did not have a place for my mother to stay.

I had invited Hattie and my mother to a pre-celebration dinner at Olive Garden. While we were eating our delicious entrée, my mother had begun to massage her chest. She complained of heartburn and a sharp, shooting pain. I had taken some Rolaids out of my purse and told my mother to take two of them.

"Here Mom, chew on these Rolaids. They will make you feel better."

My mother had taken the tablets and immediately felt much better. She began to smile, "Thank you for the relief. You are a life saver."

I handed my mother the remainder of the Rolaids and instructed her to take two tablets again before she went to bed. She took the medication and told me she would follow the "doctor's orders."

That night, Hattie said my mother complained of being tired from her trip and went straight to bed. She later woke up screaming. Hattie recalled walking into the bedroom and seeing my mother on the edge of the bed. She was pale and lifeless and appeared to have a blank stare on her face. My mother was grabbing her chest with one hand and clutching her right shoulder with the other.

Hattie said to my mother, "Are you alright? What is wrong?"

"It is my chest; it hurts so bad. The pain is moving down my right arm."

"I better call Dr. Jones and 911 for some help." Hattie quickly called 911.

Hattie told the 911 dispatcher, "Mrs. Jones is not doing so well. I need some help. I think she is having a heart attack."

"What is your location?"

"It is 372 Lenox Avenue, apartment number 71."

"Stay calm. Help is on the way."

"Thank you."

Hattie next called me and informed me of my mother's condition. "Dr. Jones, the paramedics are on the way. We need you to meet us in the emergency room at the hospital."

"Hattie, what is going on?"

"It is your mother. She is not doing so well. I called 911. We need you to meet us in the emergency room at the hospital."

My mind began to race. I had lost my father six months earlier and now my mother was in danger. I quickly threw on my hospital scrubs and ran across the street to the emergency room. I waited, almost hysterically, for the ambulance.

After undergoing several tests, my mother was diagnosed with having a massive heart attack. She was then transferred to the Cardiac Intensive Care Unit. My mother's cardiologist told me it was a miracle that my mother was still alive. I was informed that ninety-nine percent of the blood to my mother's heart was blocked. It was the worst blockage that any of the doctors had seen in a patient who was still breathing. I still have a hard time believing the words, "Your mother has suffered a massive heart attack." I was in a state of disbelief. All I could think of was the fact that my father had died just six months earlier. This could not be happening to my mother. I could not lose her too. I just couldn't believe what was happening.

The cardiologist soon recommended that my mother undergo open heart surgery. I pleaded with the cardiologist to try angioplasty and to place a stent to keep the blood vessel open. However, he reminded me that angioplasty is risky. The blood clot in my mother's heart could be shattered and move downstream. If the clot were to move, the heart could be damaged permanently. At best, angioplasty would just be temporary. At worst, it could be life-threatening. He reminded me that when it comes to open heart surgery, every minute counts.

I understood the viewpoint of the cardiologist. I knew angioplasty in this case was experimental. I realized I was taking a chance with my mother's life. However, if angioplasty was a success, then my mother's life would be spared. The recovery from angioplasty is much better, and the quality of life is much improved.

I said to myself, "It is a huge gamble. I know it is risky. I am trying to hit a three-point shot from midcourt. If I lose, the unthinkable will happen. It will be the second family funeral in six months."

I told myself over and over, "My mother cannot die. She is strong, we can beat this."

I pleaded with the cardiologist. What could be worse than cracking my mother's chest open and operating on her heart? The heart is the life force of the entire body.

♦♦♦♦♦♦♦♦♦♦♦♦♦♦♦♦♦♦♦♦♦♦♦♦♦♦♦

I take a deep breath as the tears continued to fall. Another bad memory rears it's ugly head. A few months later, my mother was fighting breast cancer. I had been so concerned with her heart condition that I never questioned her about her yearly mammogram results. I just assumed that with all the doctors' appointments, at least one appointment was for a mammogram.

Breast cancer is the most common cancer among women in the United States and is the second leading cause of death for women living in the US. The number one cause of death is still lung cancer. The lifetime risk of developing breast cancer is one in eight in persons over the age of seventy years old.[10]

A mammogram can detect a cancer the size of a pinhead. By the time the cancer is 2 centimeters (size of a dime), it has been present for more than eleven years. A mammogram is life-saving. It can identify a mass that you cannot feel at least three years before it can be detected by physical examination.[10]

How could I miss asking my mother about her mammogram results? I am an OB/GYN physician. I specialize in women's health. How could I miss something as important as the need to have regular mammograms? I forced myself to stop thinking these thoughts.

God is definitely in the miracle healing business. The cardiac angioplasty with stent placement was a success, and my mother is a one-year *breast cancer survivor*.

I look up at my mother. "Mom I have to run, I don't want to be late. No matter how bad things appear to be. I don't want to be late."

"You better get going."

"Mom, do you have anything special to do today?"

"I have an appointment at Mercy General Hospital this morning to have all my blood work drawn for my breast cancer chemotherapy treatment tomorrow. Tomorrow is my last dose of chemotherapy. Yippee! I cannot wait. Tomorrow Nurse Maria said I get to graduate. On graduation day, Maria usually brings in a cake, and we have a nice little celebration. It has been a whole year since I got the news of being diagnosed with breast cancer. Look at me now. I am a BCS—Breast Cancer Survivor."

"Mom, is Mrs. Penny coming by to take you to the hospital?"

"No, I am just having my blood work drawn so I can drive myself. Penny will take me to the hospital tomorrow."

The telephone rings.

"Penny we were just talking about you. What? I don't believe it, she was in church yesterday and was singing in the choir. She had a heart attack when she got home? That is the same way Mrs. Berry Mae Anderson died last week. Heart disease is terrible, and it is killing so many people. I hear more and more women are dying of heart disease. Yes, the doctors say my heart is doing fine. I am trying the best I can with this diet and exercise program. I plan to be here a good, long time. I have to keep Chandra straight."

I interrupt my mother's phone conversation.

"Mom, I'm going to work. Call me later and maybe, if I finish early, I can treat you to lunch at the cafeteria."

"I want you to save your money so you can buy the two new forty-two-inch plasma flat-screen television sets. Remember, they will help me with my eye strain."

"Here we go again with the eye strain story."

The cell phone rings... saved by the cell phone.

"Yes, I saw the news. I am on my way out the door; I will call you from the car."

I kiss my mother on the forehead. "Bye, Mom, got to run. I will call you later."

I collect my things and then dash out the door. I realize my operating room shoes are still inside the house. I turn around to go and get them.

"Forgotten something?"

"Yes, I forgot my operating room shoes."

I grab my shoes and leave the house.

Chapter 9

Driving to the Hospital

As I open the door of the garage, I hear thunder. I cannot believe it. The weatherman said that there was a ten percent chance of rain. As I back out of the driveway, I see the rain falling like large drops of round crystals. I know the traffic will be horrible. People around here cannot drive when the ground is dry, and I shudder to think about the traffic when the road is wet.

I turn on the radio and flip through the stations. I pause when I hear the words "special announcement."

"It is now confirmed; the OB/GYN staff at Mercy General Hospital will leave the hospital today at 8:00 a.m. I repeat, the hospital staff at Mercy General Hospital will leave the hospital today at 8:00 a.m. We are told that the hospital has just been placed on diversion. That means, if you are pregnant, do not go to Mercy General Hospital. I repeat, do not go to Mercy General Hospital. The hospital is open only for extreme emergencies. All non-emergency cases are being routed to other facilities. You can go to Broadway Memorial Hospital downtown or to University Hospital up the street. But, I repeat, the obstetrics department at Mercy General Hospital is closing today at 8:00 a.m. If you are pregnant, do not go to Mercy General Hospital."

As I change the station, I hear the same announcement: "Mercy General Hospital is closing today at 8:00 a.m. If you are pregnant, do not go to Mercy General Hospital. I repeat, if you are pregnant do not go to Mercy General Hospital."

The drive to the hospital feels like it takes an eternity in the pouring rain. I catch every red light, and I seem to be behind the slowest drivers in town. My thoughts start racing. I try to process the events of the morning, but nothing seems to make any sense. A strike! How could I be walking into such a Pandora's box? The worst part of it all, is that I am completely in the dark. I say to myself, "For better or worse I have to deal with it. I just have to find someone to tell me the truth. I hope that Charles is still at the hospital. I know he'll tell me the truth. That's it. I just have to find Charles and talk to him."

    I pull into the doctors' parking lot, and I see at least 200 people standing in front of the hospital doors. I can tell the situation is getting worse. Earlier this morning, just a handful of people were standing near the camera; now it's a serious mob. I see four police cars pull up to the hospital doors, and the crowd begins to disperse. This is a good time for me to make a quick dash into the hospital. I collect my things and head for the doors.

Chapter 10

Hospital Entrance

As I walk closer to the hospital entrance, I get a strange feeling. It is a mixture of emotions. Part of me is saying *welcome back* the other part is saying *you'd better run away*. Either way, it is strange and uncomfortable. I soon hear a familiar voice from the crowd. It is Charles.

"Chandra, is that you? I can't believe it. You have really grown up since high school."

"Thanks, Charles, I will take that as a compliment; life's been good."

"Chandra, how have you been? I heard your mother has breast cancer. How is she doing?"

"My mother was diagnosed with breast cancer last year. I am glad to report that she is doing well. You know my mom. She has a spirit that is just beating this breast cancer like a champion."

"Good to hear that. How is the rest of the family?"

"The rest of the family is also doing well."

"I have some good news. My wife's expecting our first baby. I'll be a father in two months. My wife and I have been trying so hard to have our first baby. We saw so many medical specialists. Just when we were about to give up hope…"

I see the excitement in Charles' eyes as he says, "I can't believe the baby is almost here."

"Congratulations, my mother shared the good news with me this morning. She even recommended that I take care of your baby."

"That would be great."

"Charles, I'm a maternal-fetal medicine specialist. I only take care of women with high-risk obstetrical problems. I take care of patients with 'baby mama drama.' Sounds like you and your wife have already been through enough."

"You are certainly right."

"Charles, I would love to take care of your family, but I sure hope for your sake that everything goes well."

"I see—you're right. We don't want any problems. So far, my wife's doing well. She's seeing a midwife."

"Charles, that's good. The midwives only see low-risk patients with no problems."

"Chandra, it has really been a long time and you still look the same. How long did it take you to complete all your medical training?"

"It took seventeen long, grueling years."

"Seventeen years."

"Yes, seventeen years."

"I knew you were in school a long time, but I didn't know you were there that long. Seventeen years is a long time."

"You're telling me! It was a very long time. I was in training four years for college, four years for medical school, four years for residency training in Obstetrics and Gynecology, three years for fellowship training in maternal-fetal medicine and two years in a research fellowship training program for the National Institute of Health. Yes Charles, a total of seventeen long, grueling years and, trust me, time did not fly."

"That is a lot of dedication. I am so proud of you."

"Charles, how's your brother, Tim, and the rest of the family doing?"

"My brother and the rest of the family are well. I can't wait to tell Tim you're back in town. Won't he be jealous? He is still single. I don't think he ever got over you."

"Charles, that was a long time ago. It was a different world back then. And after the drama I went through last year, the only thing I want to think about is medicine."

"Tim still says you are the one who got away. I know sparks would fly if you both were in the same room."

Blood rushes to my face, and I begin to blush.

"Okay, enough of Tim. Tell me, what brings you back to the General?"

"I have been asked to run the transport section on Labor and Delivery. Today I am here to speak to Dr. Von. The timing looks all wrong. Looks like I have entered a war zone."

"You're right about that one. This is a war zone. I would say a zone between Pearl Harbor and Desert Storm. I don't complain; this place keeps me in business. I have job security, reporting all the drama that goes on at the General."

"Charles, for some reason I feel like I am being pulled back into the madness."

"Chandra for your sake, I hope things get better. I will keep my eyes and ears open for you. If you need anything, don't hesitate to call. I consider you family; besides, if Tim had his way, you would be my sister-in-law."

"Charles, can you tell me what's really going on at this place?"

"The conflict appears to be over this policy."

I look down at the paper in his hand and read the words: Family Center Care: New on Labor and Delivery.

Charles explains, "The administrators want to attract more insurance-paying customers, so they are allowing children under the age of five access to Labor and Delivery. The doctors say they plan to strike today at 8:00 a.m. if the administrators don't change their minds. My intelligence says the doctors are going to strike this morning."

I tell him, "Children under the age of five allowed access to Labor and Delivery means trouble."

"I believe there will be a strike because unusual things have a way of happening around here." Just then, a cameraman from Channel 8 News spots my white jacket and walks towards us.

Charles warns, "Looks like the buzzards are gathering. You better go inside before this mob attacks you."

Charles blocks the view of the camera.

"Here is my card, call me when you get a chance. Give my best to your mom. My prayers are with both of you."

"Thanks, Charles, I hope to call you soon. We have a lot of catching up to do. Congratulations again on the new baby, and give my best to Tim."

Chapter 11

Mercy General Hospital

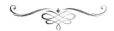

At Mercy General, people and things have a way of returning. I am a living example. Half of the staff either went to medical school or trained at this place. On the one hand, it makes for a very close group; on the other, it's like a page from the darkest nightmare. One thing is for sure, the grudges last longer than the equipment. Each grudge-match tends to get more vicious and physical as the years go by. As I walk through the hospital, I notice that very little has changed. The corridors are still dull and bleak. The air still has that musty stale medicine odor. People are scrambling everywhere. Silver metal hospital stretchers are moving like torpedoes up and down the hall. I walk up to a crowd of people who are waiting for the elevators.

A voice comes from the crowd: "Help us, help us! We have to get to Labor and Delivery. Help us, help us."

I see a pregnant lady in a wheelchair, holding a baby. She is followed by a small boy who appears very excited. Her husband tries to push through the crowd. He yells, "Move, move, my wife's in labor. Move out of the way."

The members of the crowd have plenty to say for themselves.

One bystander yells, "Give them space, let them through. Can't you see the lady is having a baby? Let them through."

The crowd begins to clear a path for the party.

Another bystander comments, "That looks like Attorney Daniel Crane."

"Sure does, I can't imagine him at this hospital. He is one of the richest lawyers around."

"Didn't Attorney Crane sue this place last year for 250 million dollars?"

"He sure did, and he won the case. He got paid 250 million big ones."

"I can't believe he's here with his pregnant wife. He must not know about the strike."

"He has to know, the strike has been plastered all over the news and on the television. I bet it even made the headlines in this morning's paper. I'm sure Attorney Crane is not living in a bubble. He has to know that the docs at Mercy General are walking out."

I say to myself, "I must be the one living in a bubble because I had no clue about all this drama." I look up at the elevators. All four are still going up.

Someone from the crowd yells, "I bet Crane is back here to sue again."

Another responds, "I heard Crane's wife delivered her last two children here at Mercy General."

"She sure did. She got sent here from big time University with both her kids."

"They say Mrs. Crane is a sickly woman. She stays more in the hospital than out."

"The Cranes might be rich, but money is not everything; it can't buy health."

"Money might not buy health, but it sure can pay for good health insurance. With good health insurance, you can pay for as much good health and pretty looks as the wallet can afford."

"You can also get replacement parts like new joints, a new liver, or a new kidney. Look at Mrs. Crane. That woman looks like she has spare parts and a new face."

The members of the crowd continue to debate Mrs. Crane's life.

"I bet Mrs. Crane stays in the hospital getting those expensive plastic surgeries. Look at her. Everything she owns is probably tucked, sucked, or cut."

"How disgusting."

"Just tell me I am wrong. Didn't you see Mrs. Crane's face? That old woman looked just like she's in her thirties. She has got to be in her late forties or early fifties. I tell you, she's been having plastic surgery."

"You're right about the insurance. My cousin Vinny had no insurance, and they took him off the breathing machine when they found out the family couldn't pay the bill. I went into Vinny's room a week later, and Vinny was gone. There was an old man on Vinny's machine, and he looked like he was loaded with money."

"Why do you say that?"

"Because next to his bed was one of those private duty nurses. She was sitting there all pretty like."

"The hospital kept your cousin on the machine for one week with no insurance. No wonder this hospital is going to pot. *You people* get too much free care."

"They don't give away the care. They keep people alive on those machines to get their organs. You know, they use people as organ donors. Where else do you think those new kidneys, livers, and other spare parts come from?"

"That can't be true. It is cheaper to get spare parts from the morgue than to keep somebody on an expensive machine for a week. Besides, I don't blame Crane for bringing his family here."

"If you find something that works, might as well stick with it."

"Looks like Crane and his kids are doing okay."

The elevator finally arrives, and the Crane party enters.

"I hope that lady and the baby make it."

"Who are you calling *You People*. Take it back, or I will ram it down your throat."

"If the shoe fits, wear it. *You People* cost the taxpayers too much money."

A fight breaks out in the crowd. Hospital security arrives, and the excitement is soon over. It takes about ten more minutes for the elevator doors to slide open. A crowd of about twenty people rush into the elevator. I follow everyone in and we stand side by side like a can of sardines. As the door starts to close, I hear a yell. A hospital employee jumps into the elevator. As the doors swing open, I see a stretcher, and then I hear a firm voice: "We have an emergency; would everyone exit the elevator. Hurry, hurry, thank you."

As we leave the elevator, I look up and see all the other elevators are going up. First the Cranes and now this. I don't have another ten minutes to waste. I decide to take the steps. Dr. Von's office is located on the seventh floor. I put on my surgical shoes. If I take my time, I know I can make it. The stairwell is musty, hot, and crowded. It appears everyone in the building has decided to go up and down the stairs. With those slow elevators, I really can't blame them.

I manage to struggle to the second floor before I get short of breath. I try to walk a little further, but chest pain sets in and my breathing gets worst. I stop on the third floor to catch the elevator.

I walk up to the crowd waiting for the next elevator. My heart is racing, and I am drenched in sweat. I don't know if it is me or this place. It is hot in this hospital year around. I believe the air conditioning unit has one setting for the temperature, and that is hot.

In the wintertime, the heat runs full blast, and in the summertime the heat runs on low. I recall how no matter how we would adjust the temperature gage, all we would get was heat coming out of the air vents. This place is a mental and physical living sauna.

I manage to make it to the seventh floor after much delay. I walk into the office, and I am greeted rather coldly by Madame Secretary Mrs. Constantine Oliver. I believe Mrs. Oliver was hired as secretary when the hospital laid the first brick. If not the first brick, I am sure she was around when the first baby was born at the General. She is a prime example of how people grow old in this place and never leave.

Mrs. Oliver looks me up and down. She slides her glasses down the tip of her nose and begins to focus on my feet. In a very sarcastic bitter tone laced with a crooked smile, she says, "Nice suit, it appears the steps got the best of you. Looks like you were no match for the steps."

She begins to laugh.

"And a good morning to you as well Mrs. Oliver. I am here to speak to Dr. Von."

"Dr. Von said to expect you this morning. Took you long enough to get here."

"Where is Dr. Von?"

"Dr. Von is in a meeting. She assigned you the office over there." Mrs. Oliver points across the room. "You can go and put your things in your office and stop breathing on me."

I walk into the office, and I notice boxes are everywhere. It looks like someone was in the process of packing but didn't quite get the chance to finish. I walk back into the main office.

"Mrs. Oliver, who left their things on top of the desk? It looks like someone was trying to pack but didn't get the opportunity to finish the job. Where can I put my personal things?"

Mrs. Oliver looks at me; she's clearly agitated. "I am just the messenger. Things around here are always changing. I don't know or care where they plan to put you. It is not clear if you will be staying in this office. For the time being, I suppose they'll find some place for you. For today, and today only, you can park your things behind my desk."

Mrs. Oliver points to a small corner next to an old, worn-out black filing cabinet that is overstuffed with papers and folders. I believe Madame Oliver actually thinks she is doing me a favor.

I look at Mrs. Oliver and say, "Where is Dr. Von? I need to talk to her as soon as possible."

"I told you, Dr. Von is in a very important administrative meeting. She's not to be disturbed. (Translation: she is unavailable to you). Haven't you been watching the news?"

It dawns on me that Dr. Von must be in a meeting regarding the hospital and the strike.

Mrs. Oliver continues, "When Dr. Von is free, I'll let her know you're looking for her." She then points again to the corner beside the file cabinet. "Dr. Jones, you can put your things there. Just know, I will not be responsible for your belongings. I won't be responsible for anything of yours that gets stolen, ransacked, or lost."

"What did you say?"

Mrs. Oliver responds, "I won't be responsible for any of your things that might get stolen, ram sacked, or lost. There have been some human-sized rats stealing things out of the offices. You know they always blame either the housekeeping staff or the secretaries. I am letting you know right now that I am not a thief. I am sure you have nothing in your belongings that would be of any interest to me anyway."

She slides her glasses back over the bridge of her nose before adding, "Even that suit looks like you bought it from an old bargain sale. Besides, it's not my style. I prefer something with a little class, style, and sophistication. You know, something with some taste."

A hospital strike and now the antics of Mrs. Oliver. This is too much.

"Morning Report starts in ten minutes. You are the Attending Physician in charge of Labor and Delivery today. Here's your pager. I put a new battery in it for you. It should work, so don't complain to me about missing your pages." She hands me the pager.

"You are officially now on the clock. You need to start moving and stop harassing me."

"Mrs. Oliver, what do you mean I'm the Attending Physician in charge of the labor deck today? I just got here. I am only here to speak to Dr. Von."

"All I have to go by is this schedule that came out late yesterday. It says that you're covering Labor and Delivery, and you're scheduled to be on call tonight."

"On call? That cannot be true!"

"You are the only doctor here today. The other doctors have walked out. Seems to me, you are the only on call candidate. I don't know what will happen the rest of the week, but for today you happen to be the only doctor around this place. So dear… you are covering Labor and Delivery and the on-call schedule."

Mrs. Oliver hands me the schedule and points to my name. I stare at the printed schedule in disbelief.

"That's you. You are Dr. Jones? We don't have another Dr. Jones in this department. That is you, isn't it?"

I take a deep breath and bite my lip. I can almost taste blood. I try my hardest to control my temper and not explode. I want to just let her have it. I need someone to vent all this pent-up aggression on and right now Mrs. Oliver is a worthy candidate. I just want to let her have it so badly.

The little voice in my head tells me, "*Calm down*. Mrs. Oliver is not worth you having a stroke from high blood pressure or a migraine headache. Just keep your cool. This woman is only trying to start a fight. You know that she's Dr. Jekyll one minute and Mr. Hyde the next. She's just a miserable old lady who likes to stir up trouble. She plans to retire soon. I only wish it was yesterday. In the meantime remember to just *calm down*. Keep your cool and try to force a smile." I can feel my temperature drop, and I begin to calm down. I even amaze myself by managing a smile.

I hear my Grandmother's wisdom: "Smile: it will keep your associates *wondering* and your adversaries *clueless*." Grandmother is definitely on target this time. Mrs. Oliver is without a clue, and she is wondering why I am smiling. Things are looking up.

I walk over to Mrs. Oliver with the widest grin I can muster. I mutter calmly through gritted teeth, "You want me to put my things where? Thank you for putting a new battery in my pager."

Mrs. Oliver's face begins to soften. Her second personality, Mr. Hyde, begins to take over.

"Dr. Jones, you can put your things right here. I will watch them for you. Your things will be safe."

I believe I'm hearing things. With Morning Report starting in a few minutes, I don't have time to figure out the antics of Madame Oliver. I place my valuables in the pocket of my lab coat and put the remainder of my belongings in the spot assigned to me by Mrs. Oliver, beside the file cabinet and a dusty old plastic pot.

On my way out of the door, I once again force myself to put on the wide grin and say, "Have a good day Mrs. Oliver." I surprise myself. My blood pressure returns to normal and I have survived round one. As I described, things are looking up.

I walk down the hall. I turn as I hear the voice of Mrs. Oliver. "Dr. Jones! Dr. Von just called. She wants you to attend the administrative meeting on the second floor. She said the meeting starts in five minutes."

Chapter 12

Administration Conference

I walk into the meeting. I see two of my former residency colleagues: my old arch rival Priscilla Coleman-Purse and semi-friend Trina Trent-Gage. I quickly take a seat next to Trina. I try very hard to avoid meeting Priscilla's gaze.

Trina welcomes me, "Chandra, it is good to see you. Too bad it has to be on a day like today."

"Good to see you, Trina. Looks like I have come to the General in the middle of a mess."

"You got that one right. This is a big mess."

Dr. Priscilla Coleman-Purse, now Chief Hospital Administrator and OB/GYN physician says, "Settle down. Settle down. It is now time to bring this conference to order."

She taps her pen on the side of her coffee cup and looks over at me with a smirk. I can almost read her mind, and it is not good. "Today is the final vote on the new Family Center Care Policy on Labor and Delivery."

Mr. Stanley Tight-Check, Chief Financial Officer, begins to hand out flyers. They read:

> Hospital For the Family:
>   Family Center Care
>   New on Labor and Delivery

All the doctors quickly take their seats and look down at the flyers. The room is composed of all the clinical decision-makers in the hospital. Each department is represented by the department chairperson. There are fourteen departments in all. Six of the doctors from the OB/GYN department, including myself and Doctors Von, Jenkins, Sullivan, Blakely, and Trent-Gage are present. The hospital attorney Donald Thigpen is also present.

Attorney Donald Thigpen addresses Mr. Tight-Check: "Stanley, I saw you on the news this morning."

"You did?"

"Yes, and it's not a good idea to swing your briefcase at the news camera, especially when you're on live television. Mercy General Hospital is in enough trouble. We don't need to be labeled as being a bunch of renegade, out-of-control administrators."

"Yeah, Yeah. I get the message. Next time no witnesses."

"*Next time* no swinging stuff at television cameras. I have enough on my plate. I don't need to have to bail you out of jail."

"Yeah, Yeah."

"If you go to jail then you'll stay in jail. This hospital will not get you out. You'll be left to your own theatrical devices and monetary discretion."

Mr. Tight-Check says sarcastically, "Whatever you say, boss man…"

Dr. Von interrupts, "I would like to address the committee."

Dr. Purse snaps, "Dr. Von, unless you have something new to tell the committee, your stalling tactics will be a waste of everyone's time. The best thing for you to do is to sit down and shut up."

Dr. Osborne (Chairman of Radiology) says, "Let her speak." Dr. Gage (Chairman of Surgery) concurs.

Dr. Von starts, "The proposal to allow children under the age of five access to Labor and Delivery is a big mistake."

Dr. Purse whines, "That's old news. We heard you say that before. Your stalling won't work. You're wasting everyone's time."

Dr. Von continues, "The proposed Family Center Care, is unsafe for all involved—the patients, staff, and visitors. I can't put my staff in jeopardy. Allowing access to underage children is unsafe, and if someone gets hurt it could ruin the hospital. I won't allow my staff to be put in danger. Our goal is to provide quality healthcare in a safe environment."

Dr. Purse and Mr. Tight-Check have their minds made up and ignore Dr. Von's comments. They don't even look at her while she's talking.

Dr. Purse declares, "Labor and Delivery needs to be brought into the twenty-first century. Our competitor, University Hospital, has a Family Center Care policy, and it's a very lucrative stream of revenue for the hospital."

Mr. Tight-Check jumps in, "University Hospital has tripled their income in twelve months while the obstetrical department at Mercy General Hospital has managed to lose money at the same rate."

Dr. Purse tells Dr. Von, "I believe you're over exaggerating this safety issue. If you and your staff do your jobs, then we won't have anything to worry about. We are bringing life back to the dead dragon—Labor and Delivery." She points at the whiteboard and reads, "This is our new advertisement—Hospital for the Family: Family Center Care: New on Labor and Delivery."

Mr. Tight-Check says authoritatively, "Time for the vote."

Administration Conference

Dr. Purse agrees, "Yes, time for the vote. This issue is now closed for discussion. Dr. Von, the committee has heard your complaints and is tired of your stalling tactics. All those in favor of the new Family Center Care Policy raise your hands."

Two-thirds of the voters raise their hands.

Dr. Purse triumphantly declares, "The vote is final. The new policy is: Hospital for the Family—Family Center Care: New on Labor and Delivery. It is now time for the next item on the agenda. All opposed can leave the meeting. You obstetricians can go."

Dr. Purse glances down at me and Doctors Jenkins, Sullivan, Blakely, and Trent-Gage.

"Dr. Von, you and your staff are free to go and try to make this hospital some money."

Mr. Tight-Check agrees, "Yeah, go and make some money."

Dr. Von says, "If this committee goes along with the Family Center Care policy, my doctors will strike. I'm warning you, Dr. Purse; my doctors will leave."

Dr. Trent-Gage adds, "Priscilla, if you enforce this Family Center Care Policy, then you can run this department by you own damn self."

Attorney Thigpen says, "Dr. Trent-Gage, you are out of line."

"Out of line, my foot. In all my years of practice, I have never seen a lawyer deliver one baby. If this policy is enforced, we're out of here. You lawyers and administrators can take over. On second thoughts, let Dr. Priscilla Purse deliver all the damn babies herself. Priscilla, I am sure you still know how to catch a baby, or has it been too long since you did some real work and got your hands dirty?"

Dr. Purse warns, "Dr. Von, put a muzzle on your stray ally */* ."

Attorney Thigpen says, "Dr. Purse and Dr. Trent-Gage that will be enough. No need to resort to such unprofessional behavior. Control yourselves."

Dr. Purse threatens further, "Dr. Von, if your doctors leave the hospital grounds today, they cannot come back." Dr. Purse gives Dr. Trent-Gage a contemptuous look. "This committee will not be held hostage by bribery or uncivilized people."

Dr. Trent-Gage replies, "Uncivilized, Priscilla? Let me show you the back of my civilized foot." Dr. Gage grabs his wife Dr. Trent-Gage by the arm.

"Calm down. Let Dr. Von handle this. You're out of line."

"Dr. Von, you tell the rest of your doctors if they strike, they will be fired. If they want to leave the hospital and continue with this strike, then they better quit, because they won't be welcomed back. If they leave, they'll be ruined."

Dr. Trent-Gage asks, "Is that a promise, wish or threat?"

"What do you think Trent-Gage?"

Dr. Von interrupts, "How do you expect me to run an OB/GYN service, the inpatient ward, outpatient offices, emergency room, consultation service, and Labor and Delivery with no physicians?"

Dr. Trent-Gage replies, "Priscilla, you have gone too far."

"Trina, we all know your problem. You're sleeping with the enemy."

"Watch it Priscilla, you have just crossed the line."

Dr. Gage interrupts, "The last time I checked, the Department of Surgery was the number one money maker for this hospital. The Departments of Obstetrics and Radiology are running a close second in generating revenue for this place."

Dr. Purse interrupts Dr. Gage, "The vote is final. The new policy is Hospital for the Family—Family Center Care: New on Labor and Delivery."

Dr. Von says, "This means trouble."

Dr. Trent-Gage adds, "This means war." Dr. Trent-Gage then storms out of the room and slams the door. She is followed by Doctors Jenkins, Sullivan, and Blakely.

My pager goes off. It is Labor and Delivery. I look up at Dr. Von.

Dr. Von tells me, "Dr. Jones, better get that. I will join you shortly."

I give her a nod and quickly exit the room.

Chapter 13

Labor and Delivery

I walk onto the Labor Ward.

Dr. Clark greets me with great enthusiasm, "Chandra, you're back. It's so good to see you. Why didn't you call me?"

I am so happy to see Charmaine Clark. We have both come a long way since our residency days. Charmaine is now the OB/GYN Residency Coordinator, and I am a Maternal Fetal Medicine Specialist. It seems like yesterday. Time sure does fly.

"Regina, what are all these little people doing in here?"

Clerk Regina points to the notice on the board that reads:

> Hospital for the Family
> Family Center Care
> New on Labor and Delivery

Dr. Clark says, "I can't believe they're really going through with this nonsense. Don't they know we plan to leave if they continue with this crazy stuff?"

Head Nurse Cynthia Simmons states, "*I* can't believe that the administrators care more about the budget than the staff."

Clerk Regina looks at the notice and then at the children, "One thing is for sure, the children are here, so what does that tell you about the dog-gone policy?"

Head Nurse Simmons adds, "Looks like money's more important than people."

"Sure is. Money buys people, and in this place it buys them cheap," says Nurse Nancy Pickens.

The clerk adds, "These little heathens are running around like they have no training at home. Just let me get a hold of just one of them. All it will take is the fear of the Lord in just one. Let me grab just one, and I'll have them all singing in the choir."

Nurse Pickens laughs, "Amen, Sister Regina, Amen."

Head Nurse Simmons asks, "Nurse Pickens, don't you have some nursely duties to perform? I know that the obstetrical triage area is full."

"On my way. I know, my place is back in the pit."

Dr. Trent-Gage slams the chart on the desk, "I could just wrap my hands around that woman's neck and strangle her. I'm not for the death penalty, but in her case I'd make an exception. This planet would be much better without the likes of Money-Bags Priscilla Coleman-Purse."

Dr. Jenkins warns, "Calm down. It's not worth getting this angry about; besides, Dr. Von will figure out something. She always does."

Dr. Blakely shrugs. "That committee has no clue of what they just did. I know Dr. Von is behind us, but this one is out of her hands."

Dr. Sullivan asks, "Trent-Gage is right. What are we going to do?"

Dr. Trent-Gage decides for the lot, "It's time to go straight to the cameras. We already have public sympathy. I saw Tight-Check on the news this morning, trying to knock down the camera man."

Dr. Jenkins laughs, "Yeah, I heard about that. It happened right in front of the hospital."

"We'll see who gets the last word. Those administrators will be sorry. Priscilla (Money Bags) Purse will pay."

Two little kids run down the hall.

"Did you see that? That little boy is not watching where he's going. It's already starting. The madness and insanity of this Family Center Care Policy are already upon us."

Clerk Regina says, "Yes, these kids have been running around all morning. All I keep saying to them is: 'Stop running! Where are your parents? Don't touch that!' I can hardly get my work done for having to babysit the rowdy bunch of crumb snatchers."

Dr. Trent-Gage notes, "This place has a curse. All it will take is for one of these kids to get hurt."

Clerk Regina interrupts, "Forget the curse. I want to know what happened in the meeting? Will there be a strike? Is this place closing down? I have a car note, mortgage, and bills to pay. Somebody tell me something. I need to know what's happening."

Dr. Trent-Gage informs her, "The policy Family Center Care passed the vote, so we're out of here. It's time for us to leave."

The poor clerk is flabbergasted, "You can't be serious. How am I gonna pay my rent? I mean, who's gonna deliver these babies and take care of these poor mothers and babies?"

"Don't know; ask Money-Bags Purse. I'm sure she has a solution. The solution just does not include us, the low… working class… citizens."

Dr. Trent-Gage grabs her bag. She turns and looks at me, "Dr. Jones, what are you going to do?"

I stare at her blankly. This is the first time I have started to process the situation. I have walked into the middle of a strike, and I have no idea what to do.

"I don't know. I just came here today to speak to Dr. Von."

"Better figure out something quick. The bullets will be flying soon, and all innocent bystanders will be expected to pick up arms or get the hell out of the way."

Dr. Clark interjects, "Trent-Gage, that is mean."

Dr. Trent-Gage retorts, "She is either for us or against us. There is no middle ground. Besides, when Money-Bags Purse gets through harassing her, she'll wish she joined our side from the beginning. Priscilla has two people on her 'I-hate-you list': Dr. Jones and Dr. Von."

Dr. Clark reminds her: "Trina that was a long time ago. The Priscilla and Jones grudge match was over twenty years ago."

Dr. Trent-Gage, ignores her, "Priscilla hates Jones. She always did and always will. You saw that *I-hate-you* look Priscilla gave to Jones when she saw her. If that was a welcome, we all will get ice water and air-conditioning in hell. Forget hell, we will get cool air in this heat box."

Dr. Trent-Gage begins to fan herself with her hand. She stares hard at me like a mad woman possessed, grabs her bag and storms out of Labor and Delivery.

Clerk Regina moans, "I can't believe this place has come to this. What are we gonna do?"

Silence engulfs the unit. We all just stare at the sign on the bulletin board. It is almost if the words can speak.

>Hospital for the Family:
>Family Center Care
>New on Labor and Delivery.

I walk over to Charmaine. "Charmaine, we need to talk. I came here today to speak to Dr. Von. When I got here, I was told by Madame Secretary Oliver that I am already covering Labor and Delivery. She also told me that I am on the on-call schedule for tonight. I just came here to speak to Dr. Von. What is going on?"

"Let's go somewhere quiet like the doctor's lounge where we can speak in private," Charmaine suggests.

The doctor's lounge is the least private place in the entire hospital. The room has an intercom speaker system that has a way of turning itself on. One night, two medical students got caught in the room making out. One of the students hit the button and everyone in the Labor and Delivery ward heard everything in full hot and steamy detail. I look at Charmaine. "It might be better to talk in the hallway than go into the lounge with the speaker system."

Charmaine begins to laugh. It is almost as if she can read my mind, "Just don't hit the speaker system, and we'll be alright." We leave Labor and Delivery and walk into the doctor's lounge.

Chapter 14

Doctor's Lounge

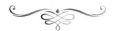

The table is covered with left-over food, and the lounge smells of musty scrubs and bloody operating shoes. The place looks like a boarding house for rodents or a breeding place for pigs. Charmaine pours herself a cup of coffee.

"Want some coffee? I can make a fresh pot." I look at the coffee pot. It has a green tinge and I am sure that some type of bacteria is currently partying inside it. I turn up my nose and shake my head.

"I forgot. You are a tea drinker; you don't drink coffee." She's right, but even if I did drink coffee, I wouldn't be able to bring myself to drink that green stuff. We both sit at the table.

"Chandra, it's bad; things are really out of control."

"Charmaine, I wish I'd had a chance to talk to you sooner. I heard that you were out of the country."

"Yes, I went home. My mother is not doing too well." "What is wrong?"

"She fell and hurt her hip, but she's doing much better now." "And how's your dad?"

"Dad's doing well. He's still preaching, taking care of mom, and running the city."

"Charmaine, tell me: what's going on around here at the General?"

"The administrators are giving us a fit. Your old buddy, Priscilla Coleman-Purse, is the ring leader."

"My old buddy? Since when were Priscilla and I ever buddies? She has hated me since internship."

"You mean since you dated Arthur and jammed her with the breech delivery."

"I dated Arthur six months after they broke up, and Priscilla jammed herself by lying about the breech delivery."

"You don't have to convince me; I was there, remember?"

"Arthur and Priscilla dated before we were even residents at this place."

"Sounds like you don't know."

"Charmaine, what are you talking about? Know what?"

"Your old buddy, Priscilla, is now married to Arthur."

"Really?"

"Yes, they got married about three years ago. She got knocked up. The kid looks nothing like Arthur. Some say it was donor sperm from who knows where. Anyway, Arthur bought the story, and he married her because of the kid."

"I can't believe it."

"I know; it shocked all of us. Broomstick Priscilla married with a kid. Yeah, shocked the hell out of all of us. During the pregnancy, she really was the drama queen: hyperemesis, diabetes, preeclampsia. We were all waiting for her to have a nervous breakdown or seizure in the bed. There was a money pool with hopes of her blowing a vessel in her brain leading to her early retirement."

"Really?"

"But you know, some people. She just came back meaner and more full of hate than ever. She just seems mad at the world."

"And now Priscilla is the chief hospital administrator."

"You got it. She is just torturing everybody."

My heart begins to flutter, and I think, "I am doomed. I have been through a living hell. Now this! I am, without a doubt, doomed." I look at Charmaine; in that moment of silence we exchange a look that words cannot express.

"Charmaine, tell me about Priscilla. I need to know the whole story."

"Priscilla stopped practicing obstetrics about five years ago. She turned in her OB hat and became the administrator."

"I bet since Priscilla stopped delivering babies, the infant death rate at the hospital has gone down."

Charmaine laughs, "Sad but true. There have been fewer babies dying in the last five years. Good for the babies but bad news for us."

It is hard to believe. Priscilla Coleman was my second-year resident when I was an intern. I dated Arthur one time, and that started the feud. The breech delivery episode was just the icing on the cake. One thing was for sure, working with Priscilla was not going to be anything close to civilized or pleasant.

"We call Priscilla, Money-Bags Purse. She's doing her darndest to take this department down. She hates all of us, but she really has it in for Dr. Von."

"Sounds like Priscilla hates someone other than me. One thing is for sure. Any enemy to Priscilla is an ally to me. Charmaine, why does Priscilla have it in for Dr. Von?"

"Dr. Von and Dr. Arthur Purse were up for the job of chairperson for the OB/GYN department last year. Dr. Purse made everyone painfully aware that he planned to become the next Chief of Staff at this hospital."

"I see, in order to be the Medical Chief of Staff, you first have to be chair of one of the departments."

"Sure do. When Dr. Von was named chair of OB/GYN, Dr. Purse went postal. At the departmental reception for Dr. Von, Dr. Purse stormed in and threw his resignation letter in Dr. Von's face. Dr. Purse ranted and raved something terrible. He swore that he would not work for a woman, and then he cursed the entire department. It was a really bad scene. I thought they were going to have to call security and escort him out of the building. Dr. Purse left the party and packed up his office. He stormed out of the hospital the same day. It was a big mess."

"Where's Arthur now?"

"He's now head of the OB/GYN department at University Hospital, our number one competitor. Too bad he did not take his wife, Priscilla, with him. This place would definitely be better off without the likes of her. That woman is pure evil. We all know that she wants revenge for her husband. The writing is on the wall."

"Charmaine, sounds like Priscilla is still up to her same tricks."

"Yes, she is. Money-Bags has been trying to destroy Dr. Von and destroy this department. We both know Priscilla hates OB. I believe that Money-Bags came up with this Family Center Care Policy out of pure hatred. She wants to see us fail, and so far she's getting her wish. It's just pure evil I tell you—pure evil."

I think of my grandmother's wisdom: "Evil comes in the form of a conspiracy or ambush" and wonder if this type of situation was what she was referring to.

"Don't the rest of the administrators know what she's doing?" I ask.

"Something is definitely wrong at this place. Everybody around here walks around with blinders on. Nobody says or does anything to stand up to Priscilla."

"What about Trina Trent-Gage? She seems to be upset about what's happening."

"Trina has not changed. She is still so fickle and wishy-washy. She doesn't know what she'll do from one day to the next."

I remember Trina during internship. She had a quiet disposition, but when she got upset, she was a loaded pistol. I recall the time she and Priscilla got into a fight in the on-call room. Priscilla was always picking on us interns, and that day Trina snapped and jumped on Priscilla. We let them fight for about ten minutes before pulling them apart. Trina kicked Priscilla's butt. Following the fight, Priscilla started doing nice things for Trina. In a twisted sort of sense, the two almost became friends. One day they would be speaking, the next day they would be at each other's throats, going for the jugular. With Priscilla, one never knew which way the ball was bouncing. However; when it came to me, all bets were off. Priscilla hated me, and she made sure everybody knew it.

Charmaine confirmed, "We can't depend on Trina."

"Charmaine, tell me about the strike. How did it come to this?"

"That was Trina's idea. We have no choice. If we stay and something happens to one of the children, we can get sued and lose our medical licenses. So what choice do we have? You remember what happened to that kid who got run over by a stretcher in residency? It was only by the grace of God that he wasn't seriously injured."

"Yes, I remember."

"Chandra, what are you going to do? If you stay, you'll be the only doctor here."

"I don't know."

"If you stay, you will be type-cast and labeled a traitor."

"I know."

"If you leave, Priscilla will hang you. On second thoughts, Priscilla will hang you if you leave or torture you if you stay."

I contemplate my situation. Charmaine is right. If I join the strike, I will be playing right into Priscilla's hands, but if I stay, life with Priscilla will be miserable. This is a no-win situation. I am damned if I do and damned if I don't. And just when I thought things could not get worse.

"I suppose Dr. Von will be here with you. She'll probably be your only backup. The rest of us are walking out."

The speaker in the lounge goes off, and we hear Clerk Regina paging me, "Dr. Jones, are you in there?"

"Yes."

"You're needed on Labor and Delivery right away."

"Thanks, here I come. Charmaine, we'll have to finish this later. For now, I will have to stay here and cover Labor and Delivery. I need to speak to Dr. Von."

Charmaine walks over to the automated machine where the scrubs are kept. She punches in her code. The door opens, "You still wear a size extra small?"

"No, I have moved up to a size small. Thank you very much." Charmaine begins to laugh. She pulls out two pairs of size small scrubs.

"Since you're going to be the only doctor at the hospital today, you better change into scrubs. Go ahead and change in the locker room. I'll find out what the problem is on Labor and Delivery."

"Thanks, Charmaine."

I walk into the locker room and quickly change my clothes. I look down at my feet. Thank goodness I have my trusty operating room shoes on. It looks like it is going to be a long twenty-four-hour shift, and this is just the beginning of my life at the General.

Charmaine yells into the locker room, "Chandra, it is time for Morning Report. You go to report; I will check out things on Labor and Delivery."

Chapter 15

Morning Report

I walk into Morning Report as the last few students enter the room. The classroom is just as I remembered. There are about twenty chairs lined up against the sides of the room. An old projector is placed on the center of a long table that hugs the back wall. The projector is at least thirty years old. It did not work when I was here before, and I see it does not work now.

My cell phone rings; it's my mom, "Mom, where are you?"

"I'm sitting in the cafeteria waiting for you. I just finished my chemotherapy and need a ride home."

"Waiting on me? What are you talking about?"

"There was a vacancy in the chemo schedule, so I was able to get my last treatment today. My head is a little woozy. I need a ride home."

"Mom, I'm tied up in Morning Report. We're just getting started. I should be able to break free in about thirty minutes. Just have some breakfast; I will be there as soon as I can."

"That's okay, dear. I'll call Penny. She'll come and take me home."

"Mom it should not be that long."

"I am not feeling too well, and I need to go home and lay down. I will just call Penny to come and get me."

"Okay, Mom. Call me back if you can't reach Mrs. Penny or call me when you get home."

"Okay, dear. I'll call you back."

I look at the residents.

"My name is Dr. Jones. I am the new Attending. Time to get started." The screen covering the board is slowly lifted. It makes a loud, piercing noise like someone running their nails along a chalkboard. It gives me chills just hearing that sound: *Sqreeeeeeeeeeech!*

I see an old plastic flowering plant. It is covered with dust and housed in a large ceramic pot. The plant was given to one of the resident doctors on Labor and Delivery as a gift during my former stint at the General. I still don't know how it found a home in this room but, for some strange reason, it is still here.

I survey the room. All the people in the room are trainees. They have no history and are bright with enthusiasm. Their lives have not yet been tainted. I remember sitting in those same seats. Time has a way of building armor.

Dr. Charles Cates is the chief resident covering the obstetrical service. I remember those days, and I don't want them to return. I have heard that Resident Cates is a good chief resident. He is attentive to details and runs the OB service as if he is a commando in the Marines. He might be tough with his colleagues, but he is well liked by the patients and staff. I am sure that having sophisticated good looks with a baritone bedroom voice does not hurt his appeal.

Chief Resident Cates walks to the front of the room and begins to speak. "Quiet down, everyone. Time to do the rounds on the patients on Labor and Delivery. Dr. Blake, you can start."

Dr. Brian Blake is a second-year resident. He opens, "Room 1 is Mrs. Thompson. She presented last night in active labor. This is her third pregnancy, and it's her second child. Last check, she was six centimeters. She's now requesting an epidural for pain control. Her first child was eight pounds. This baby is seven pounds and some change. A side note: she has a very mean mother-in-law. The mother-in-law keeps yelling at Mrs. Thompson and tells her to suck up the pain and take it like a woman. Some serious social dynamics are going on in that room. Don't want to be a fly on the wall when that baby makes the grand entrance."

The medical students begin to laugh.

Resident Blake continues, "Room 2 is Mrs. Hope. She presented last night in labor with triplets. She just had twins last year."

Dr. Cates interrupts, "Dr. Blake time to let the students present the new patients." Morning Report seems to be dragging on.

Chapter 16

Mother's Accident

My mother picks up the cell phone and calls Mrs. Penny.

"Penny, can you come to Mercy General Hospital and pick me up?"

"I'm at University Hospital with Sam. He just went in the doctor's office. As soon as Sam is finished, I'll swing by and pick you up."

"That's okay, Penny. I talked to Barbara earlier. She's home today. I'll call her. I'm sure she'll come and get me."

"Okay, but if Barbara can't take you home, call me back."

"Thanks, Penny."

The sickness returns and Mother starts to feel worse. She says to herself, "I must go home and lay down. I can make it. I don't live that far from the hospital. I have to get out of here. I know I can make it."

Mother leaves the cafeteria and the hospital. She is still under the influence of the IV sedation. After walking around in circles, she manages to find her car, which is parked in the front of the hospital in one of the handicap spots. She gets into the car and tells herself, "I can make it. I can make it home by myself." Mother fumbles with the car keys and has trouble attaching her seat belt. She gets frustrated and decides to drive off. Two blocks away from the house, Mother starts to feel sick again. She bends over to throw up and does not notice the upcoming light is red.

◆◆◆◆◆◆◆◆◆◆◆◆◆◆◆◆◆◆◆◆◆◆◆◆◆◆

Mrs. Karen Johnson sees the car speeding through the light, but it is too late for her to stop. She swerves to the right. The Johnson car is struck on the driver's side. The car begins to crumble. Both of the front airbags immediately deploy. A third car comes speeding behind Mrs. Johnson. It is unable to stop. The car strikes the Johnson car from the back. John Rolston pulls his car over to the right. He has just witnessed the entire episode. He grabs his cell phone and calls 911: "I need help. There's an accident on 10th and Pine. It involves three cars."

The operator asks, "Is anyone injured?"

John gets out of his car. "I don't know, the accident just happened. It looks bad. Three cars are involved. We need help."

"I will send help right away."

Chapter 17

Emergency Services

Police officers Kelly and Bruce arrive on the scene. They are joined by Paramedic Team 56 and Paramedic Team 72. Officer Kelly and Paramedic Team 56 (Paula and Todd) rush to the car of Mrs. Johnson and her two daughters. Officer Bruce and Paramedic Team 72 (Jason and Vance) rush to the car of Mrs. Jones. Police officers Still and Beckworth also arrive on the scene.

◆◆◆◆◆◆◆◆◆◆◆◆◆◆◆◆◆◆◆◆◆◆◆◆◆◆◆

Mother's Car

Officer Bruce opens the car door, "I need help over here." Officer Bruce struggles to free my mother from her vehicle. She is not wearing her seat belt, and it is unclear as to whether she hit her head on the steering wheel. She is gently removed from her vehicle and quickly placed in the ambulance.

Paramedic Jason tells his partner, "We need to go to the General. Better step on it. This lady is not doing so good."

Vance replies, "Isn't the General on strike?"

"Only for pregnant patients. This woman's not pregnant. Better get going."

Paramedic Vance turns on the siren, and they are off to Mercy General Hospital.

◆◆◆◆◆◆◆◆◆◆◆◆◆◆◆◆◆◆◆◆◆◆◆◆◆◆◆

Johnson Car

Officer Kelly walks over to the Johnson car. He sees an adult female in the driver's seat and two children in the back seat.

Officer Kelly radios, "I need help over here. I got a lady trapped by the airbag and two kids trapped in the back seat."

The girls are screaming hysterically.

"Mrs., Can you hear me?"

"Yes, I can hear you, but I can't move. The air bag is crushing my chest. It's hard to breath."

"Ma'am, what is your name?"

"My name is Karen Johnson."

"Mrs. Johnson, we will get you and the girls out of the car. Just hold on." "I'm pregnant. I need help with my baby."

Paramedic Todd bends down close to the window, "Ma'am did you say you're pregnant?"

"Yes, and it is hard to breathe."

Officer Kelly is unable to open the door from the driver's side.

"Hold on Mrs. Johnson."

Fire Rescue Squad members Baxley and Dustin walk over to the car.

Officer Kelly tells them, "I need help getting this pregnant lady out of the car. The door on her side is jammed, and she's trapped by the air bag."

Baxley says, "Dustin, go and get the deflator out of the truck."

Paramedic Todd calls the station, "We need more backup."

The operator asks, "What is the situation?"

"I have two children that need to be transported to the hospital and a pregnant patient trapped in the car."

"Help is on the way."

Paramedic Todd then asks Mrs. Johnson, "Ma'am are you injured? Can you feel your baby moving?"

Mrs. Johnson starts to cry, "My baby's not moving. I'm having trouble breathing. It's hard to talk."

"Ma'am, I need you to stay calm for your sake and that of your baby."

"My girls are in the back seat. My girls need help."

The Fire Rescue Squad removes the back door from the Mrs. Johnson car. The girls are gently lifted from the back seat. Both girls are given oxygen via face mask. The girls are quickly placed in the ambulance and taken to Mercy General Hospital.

The Fire Rescue Squad next removes the front door of Mrs. Johnson's car and deflates the air bag. Mrs. Johnson is pulled carefully from the car. Todd does a quick assessment.

Mrs. Johnson is in a critical condition.

Todd calls to his partner, Paula: "Call the dispatcher at Mercy General Hospital! Let them know that we have to transport a pregnant patient because she's critical."

Paula reminds him, "We can't take the patient to Mercy General. The hospital is on diversion."

Emergency Services

"I know, but this lady and baby will die if we don't get them to the closest hospital."

Paula quickly goes to the truck. She picks up the radio and calls Mercy General Hospital: "This is Paramedic Team 56 responding to an accident on 10th and Pine. We have a critical patient, and she looks like she is eight months pregnant."

The dispatcher says, "Mercy General Hospital is on diversion for all obstetrical patients. Patients are to be diverted to University Hospital or Bayside Memorial. I repeat Mercy General Hospital is on diversion. All pregnant patients are to be diverted to University Hospital or Bayside Memorial."

"University Hospital is ten miles away, and Bayside Memorial is twenty miles away in the opposite direction."

Dispatcher: "Just relaying the message."

"In this traffic we are looking at a thirty-minute delay in treatment. This lady cannot afford that."

"I repeat, Mercy General Hospital is on diversion for all OB patients. We cannot accept any obstetrical transports at this time. You can transfer the patient to University Hospital or Bayside Memorial. The choice is yours. I repeat, Mercy General Hospital is not accepting any OB patients. This hospital is closed for OB because we have no doctors."

"We have to bring the patient to you Mercy General. There's no time. This lady has no other options."

"You're going to have to speak to the ER Attending."

Paula begins to shout, "Fine... Let me speak to the doctor. This lady is critical; we need some help!"

"Stop shouting and hold for the doctor."

Overhead page: "Dr. Carter you're needed for emergency triage call in the dispatching area. Dr. Carter emergency triage call in the dispatching area."

Dr. Carter walks into the Emergency Medicine dispatching area. "What is the problem?"

"Crazy paramedic on the line. She has an OB emergency. Will not take no for an answer. She just keeps shouting. She wants to bring a pregnant patient to Mercy General. Told her no docs are here."

"This is Dr. Carter at Mercy General Hospital. How can we help you?"

"This is Paramedic Team 56 responding to an accident on 10th and Pine. We have a critical patient who appears to be eight months pregnant. Mercy General, you're the closest hospital. We have no choice. We have to bring her to you."

"I understand. How soon will you be here?"

"Estimated arrival time is ten minutes."

"Okay, transfer accepted."

"Thank you."

Paula walks back over to Todd. They place Mrs. Johnson in the ambulance. Paula gives Mrs. Johnson oxygen by bag ventilation. Todd gets behind the wheel. He then looks back in the ambulance at Paula and Mrs. Johnson.

"Hold on Paula, we're off to Mercy General Hospital." They quickly leave with the lights flashing.

The dispatcher informs Dr. Carter, "We have three other victims arriving from the same motor vehicle accident. One elderly female and two children. It sounds like it was a bad wreck."

Dr. Carter orders, "I need to speak with the Attending on Labor and Delivery."

Chapter 18

Morning Report

We have been in this small stuffy room for about fifty minutes, listening to every detail of every patient. The new students are presenting the patients, and it is torture. The students have to learn, so I try to stay attentive and make the best of it.

Just then, the four trauma pagers go off one after the next.

Chief Resident Cates says, "This sounds serious. I'd better call Labor and Delivery to see what all the commotion is about." He walks to the corner of the room where the hospital phone is hanging on the wall and dials Labor and Delivery.

"Dr. Cates here, responding to the trauma pages."

Clerk Regina tells him, "The ER wants to speak to the Attending."

Chief Resident Cates turns and says, "Dr. Jones, Labor and Delivery want to speak to you." Resident Cates hands me the telephone.

"Hello, this is Dr. Jones."

Clerk Regina says, "Dr. Jones, we need you right away. Dr. Carter called from the Emergency Room... said he needs to talk to the Attending... said page you 911... sounds serious."

I tell Chief Resident Cates and second-year Resident Blake to follow me to Labor and Delivery. The rest of the team is instructed to go to the clinic. As we leave the classroom and enter the hallway, the team is joined by Dr. Marcus Green (anesthesiologist) and his resident. The trauma pagers go off again.

Dr. Green says, "Good to see you Dr. Jones. Have you any idea what's causing all this commotion?"

"I don't know, but it sounds like trouble in the emergency room."

Dr. Green tells me, "I was told a motor vehicle accident patient is in route. What's going on with Labor and Delivery? I thought we were on diversion because of the strike?"

"We are on diversion, and I don't know what the status of my labor ward is today. We already have more patients than beds; it does not look good."

Chapter 19

Labor and Delivery

The team enters Labor and Delivery.
Dr. Green asked incredulously, "What are these little people doing in here?"
Clerk Regina points to the bulletin board:

> Hospital for the Family
> Family Center Care
> New on Labor and Delivery.

Dr. Green asks, "That starts today?"
The clerk replies, "It certainly does, and we're being overtaken by little alien people."
Dr. Clark says to me, "Chandra, I held down the fort for you. You guys were in Morning Report a long time. The new students must have been presenting." We look at each other and smile.
"Charmaine you are right, some things never change. Student presentations are still long and involve complex patient histories."
"The ER just called. I don't know what is happening. Better call them back."
"Regina, any word from the emergency room?"
"No, not yet."
"Regina, contact the ER for me. I need to speak to Dr. Carter."
Clerk Regina picks up the phone and calls the ER. I walk down the hall and into Labor Room 6. As I enter the room, I see children jumping up and down in the chairs. They are out of control.
"Hello, my name is Dr. Jones. I am the Attending Physician on Labor and Delivery today. We have a few emergencies on the labor ward. We would appreciate it if you keep

all children under parental supervision and in this room for their safety. We don't want children to get hurt in the hallway. Thank you for your cooperation."

The father tells his children, "Stop jumping on the chairs and sit your butts down. Don't have me pull off my belt."

I think to myself, "Just what the doctor ordered." I leave the room and then walk back to the front desk. Clerk Regina calls the ER, "Hello, this is Labor and Delivery."

ER Clerk Evilyna answers, "ER Hold."

All seven Emergency Room telephone lines are ringing at the same time.

ER Clerk Evilyna continues to answer the telephone lines, "ER Hold… ER Hold… ER Hold." She returns to the telephone line with Clerk Regina, "ER, who are you holding for?"

"This is Labor and Delivery, and I am holding for Dr. Carter. Dr. Jones, the Labor and Delivery Attending, is waiting to talk to Dr. Carter."

"Why didn't you say that in the first place? Dr. Carter is right here."

"I tried to but…"

She is interrupted by Dr. Carter, "This is Dr. Carter."

"This is Labor and Delivery. Dr. Carter, Dr. Jones wants to speak to you."

"Dr. Jones, Dr. Carter on line four." I pick up line four.

"Hello, this is Dr. Jones."

"Dr. Jones, I have just been informed by the paramedics that a motor vehicle accident patient is on route. She's approximately eight months pregnant and is in critical condition. There's no word on the status of her baby. The patient should be here any moment."

"Dr. Carter, Labor and Delivery is on diversion. I'm sure you're aware that the OBs are on strike."

"I know, but Mercy General is the closest hospital. The mother is critical. I had no choice but to accept the transfer."

"We'll just have to make the best of it. My team will be ready. Call me again when the patient arrives."

As soon as Dr. Carter hangs up the telephone, Mrs. Johnson is rushed through the doors. She is escorted by Paramedics Paula and Todd.

Chapter 20

Emergency Room

Paramedic Todd reports to Dr. Carter, "This is the pregnant patient who was involved in the motor vehicle accident. She was conscious at the scene but is now unresponsive."

"Take her to Trauma Room 3."

Mrs. Johnson is quickly taken to Trauma Room 3 and transferred onto the trauma bed. Dr. Carter says, "1, 2, 3, LIFT!"

Paramedic Paula continues to provide oxygen via a face mask.

Resident Doctor Vicks quickly listens to the lungs for the sound of breathing. Dr. Carter shines the pen light in Mrs. Johnson's eyes. Resident Doctor Stevens pulls out the ultrasound machine to look at the baby.

Resident Vicks says, "Breathing sounds are diminished bilaterally."

Resident Stevens reports, "The baby's moving and has a good heartbeat. The leg measures 32 weeks."

Dr. Carter interjects, "Pupils are equal and reactive to light."

Resident Vicks gives Mrs. Johnson a sternal rub. There is a mild response. Mrs. Johnson is simultaneously placed on the monitors.

Dr. Carter asks, "Mrs. Johnson, can you hear me?"

Mrs. Johnson opens her eyes and nods her head.

"Mrs. Johnson, do you feel your baby moving?"

"No."

"Mrs. Johnson, do you know what happened?"

"No."

"Mrs. Johnson, you're at Mercy General Hospital. You were in a car accident. Do you remember anything about the accident?"

Mrs. Johnson closes her eyes.

Dr. Carter looks up at the monitor.

Dr. Carter says, "Blood pressure low, heart rate and respiration up."

Resident Vicks asks, "Do you want to intubate?"

"Not yet. We can hold off intubation for now. She needs more fluids. Start another IV and place a Foley catheter."

Head Nurse Kelly Anderson asks, "What type of labs do you want, Dr. Carter?"

"I want a type and screen, chemistry profile, complete blood count, and a urine analysis."

Nurse Kilpatrick places the Foley catheter, "I see blood down here."

Resident Stevens says, "Dr. Carter, she's bleeding. Better get her upstairs."

Dr. Carter asks, "How's the baby?"

Resident Stevens looks with the ultrasound machine again. "Baby looks the same. I don't feel any contractions."

Dr. Carter looks at Paramedic Todd and asks, "Any other history on the patient?"

Paramedic Todd answers, "No, nothing else. She has been pretty much out of it."

Dr. Carter instructs, "Nurse Kelly, check and see if she has a medical record here at this hospital. Get Dr. Jones from Labor and Delivery on the phone. I want to send Mrs. Johnson upstairs right away."

Head Nurse Anderson puts the blood and urine specimens in a bag and walks up to the front desk, "Clerk Evilyna, I need you to send these specimens off to the lab, stat. Dr. Carter wants to speak to Dr. Jones on Labor and Delivery. Transfer the call back to Trauma Room 3 when the call comes in."

The clerk asks, "How am I gonna send off those unlabeled specimens? No one gave me any information about that patient. Her details are not in the computer, and I don't have a hospital ID number on her. I can't send off specimens without labels or an ID number." She smacks her lips and rolls her eyes at Head Nurse Anderson, "What do you expect me to do? Make up a number just cause you put those specimens in front of me?"

Head Nurse Anderson says, "Do the best you can."

ER Clerk Evilyna asks, "Where is the ambulance triage form?"

Head Nurse Anderson places the ambulance triage form on the counter next to the specimens, "I don't have time for this right now, Evilyna. Check the medical records to see if the patient has an old chart here at this hospital. Dr. Carter wants to speak to the OB Attending. Get Dr. Jones on the telephone and transfer the call back into Trauma Room 3." She walks back into Trauma Room 3, grumbling to herself, "Someone is going to hurt that woman in one day. She's an accident waiting to happen. The sooner, the better."

ER Clerk Evilyna calls Labor and Delivery.

Clerk Regina answers the phone, "Labor and Delivery, how can I help you?"

"Dr. Carter wants to speak to Dr. Jones about a patient in the Emergency Room."

"What patient?"

"Accident patient."

"Does the patient have a name?"

"I don't want to speak to you. I said, 'Dr. Carter wants to speak to Dr. Jones.' I'm busy down here, and you're wasting my time. Put Dr. Jones on the *%#* phone."

Clerk Regina looks at the phone, "If I wasn't a Christian woman I would tell her a thing or two. In the old days, I would have cussed her out and enjoyed it. She better really be glad that I've changed."

Clerk Regina uses the overhead paging system:

> *"Dr. Jones to nursing station."*
> *"Dr. Jones to nursing station."*
> *"Dr. Jones call from Emergency Room."*

I walk up to the nursing station. "Regina, what line is the ER on?"

"Dr. Carter is on line two."

"Hello, this is Dr. Jones."

"Motor Vehicle Accident patient is here. Mother has some vaginal bleeding. I want to send her up to you right away."

"Okay, we'll be expecting her."

I hang up the telephone and look at Head Nurse Simmons, "Mrs. Simmons, the patient in the motor vehicle accident is here. She's on her way from the emergency room. The report from Dr. Carter sounds like the patient may need surgery. I want her to go in the labor room next to the operating room."

She replies, "Labor Room 8 is available."

"Thanks. Time to mobilize the team. The patient will be here any moment."

Chapter 21

Catastrophe

Attorney Daniel Crane is waiting on Labor and Delivery for Resident Doctor Saunders to complete the assessment on his wife, Mrs. Sheila Crane. Attorney Crane is having a difficult time controlling his two sons. Michael (Micky) is three years old, and Christopher (Chris) is eleven months old. "Micky, stop running around this room and keep your hands off the machines," Crane orders.

Micky has the natural curiosity of a three-year-old child and is full of energy. He is particularly interested in the fetal monitor with the moving paper. The paper fascinates him so much that he tries to pull it out of the machine.

"Micky, leave that paper and machine alone. I want you to be good. If you continue to misbehave, Mom and I will have to leave you here at the hospital all by yourself."

Micky looks up at his father innocently with his big brown eyes, "Okay, Dad, Micky be good. Micky will be a good boy."

Baby Christopher begins to cry.

Mrs. Crane says, "Honey, there's a bottle in my bag. I think Chris is hungry. It is past his feeding time." Attorney Crane walks over to where his wife's bag is placed. He finds the bottle and starts to feed Chris. Micky takes advantage of his father's lack of attention and begins to pull the paper out of the machine again.

Resident Saunders says, "Mrs. Crane, it is a false alarm. Your cervix is closed. You're not in labor. The contractions are already starting to space out. You have had one contraction in the last twenty minutes."

"Another case of false labor? I was so sure my cervix was starting to open. Those contractions were really strong earlier. I guess I waited too late to come to the hospital."

"Mrs. Crane, it is false labor. The contractions you were having are called Braxton Hicks contractions. They normally go away after you get IV fluids."

"Why did my contractions stop with the IV fluids?"

"The fluids trick the brain and stop false contractions."

"So that's why the doctors always say drink plenty of fluids?"

"Yes, you're right. So go home and continue to drink water. We want you to drink a gallon of water a day."

"A gallon of water? That is a lot of water to drink. There is no way I can drink all that."

"It may sound like it's a lot of water, but if you continually sip on water throughout the day you can drink a gallon with no problem. The key is to remember to keep water with you at all times. When you watch television, continue to keep drinking water. When a commercial comes on television, grab your water and take a sip. More importantly, when you leave home, make sure you have some water with you."

"The more I drink, the more I have to go to the bathroom. This baby is pushing on my bladder. With the extra fluids, I will just be more miserable. My body can't take much more of this."

"Mrs. Crane you might be miserable right now, but remember, your baby is premature. You are only twenty-three weeks pregnant. If your baby is born today, it will not survive. You have to be twenty-four weeks for the baby to have a chance of survival. I'm sure that you don't want to deliver a baby that has health problems."

Attorney Crane agrees, "Honey, look on the bright side. We both know how you hate needles. If you drink plenty of water, you won't have to come to the hospital for a false-alarm check."

"Dr. Saunders, how can I be sure that I am drinking enough water?" asks Mrs. Crane.

"If your urine looks like water, you're consuming enough fluids. It is that simple. What goes in should look like what comes out."

"I take those prenatal vitamins, and they turn my urine dark yellow."

"That is true, but if you're drinking enough water, after the second void of the morning, the urine will start to turn clear."

"Thank you, Dr. Saunders. I promise to do better."

"You are welcome, Mrs. Crane. I will give you a prescription to help you rest when you get home."

Resident Saunders then turns to Attorney Crane who is still having a time controlling his two sons, Micky and Chris, "Your wife is cleared to go home. I'd like for her to follow-up with her doctor in two days."

I walk into the Labor Room.

"Resident Saunders, is everything okay in here?"

"Yes, Dr. Jones. I am discharging Mrs. Crane."

"We have an emergency coming up from the ER. We need you on deck."

"Be right there Dr. Jones."

I leave the room.

"Mrs. Crane, do you have any questions?" asks Resident Saunders.

"No doctor, thank you for the information."

Mrs. Crane then turns to her husband, "Honey, will you take the boys outside the room and wait for me while I get dressed?"

"Sure honey, we'll be right outside the door." Attorney Crane collects all their belongings. He then escorts Micky and Chris out of the room. The three of them wait for Mrs. Crane right outside the labor room door.

Head Nurse Simmons approaches Attorney Crane, "Sir, would you please wait for your wife in the waiting room?"

"My wife will only be a minute. She's just getting dressed, and we'll all be leaving very soon."

"I understand Sir, but we're very busy, and we cannot have family members standing in the hallway. Please take your family and wait for your wife in the family waiting area." Micky takes advantage of his father's preoccupation with Head Nurse Simmons and makes a clean getaway down the hall.

I am standing at the corner of the nursing station as the little boy escapes from his father and runs by.

"Okay, nurse, we'll wait for my wife in the family waiting area."

"Thank you, Sir."

Attorney Crane then looks around and does not see his son, Micky. "Micky, where are you? Micky, where are you?" Micky is close to the large grey swinging doors. He hears his father call his name, and he stops in his tracks.

The Labor and Delivery doors swing open wide. The stretcher bearing Mrs. Johnson is pushed rapidly through the door. By the time Paramedic Paula sees the little boy, it is too late. Micky is in the direct path of the fast-moving stretcher. The stretcher cannot be stopped. Mrs. Crane opens the door. She is horrified by what she sees. Bang! Micky is hit!

Micky's tiny body is thrown into the air. He then crashes onto the Labor Room floor. The stretcher loses control and strikes the wall. All eyes are on Micky. His twisted body lies motionless, and he is making no sound.

Labor and Delivery is still. No one speaks. No one moves. Everyone is in a state of shock. The silence is broken by the piercing scream of Mrs. Crane: "Micky! My son! My son! Micky!"

Attorney Crane looks on in disbelief. Baby Christopher begins to scream.

The medical team rush to Micky's side.

Head Nurse Simmons takes action, "Regina, hit the Emergency Code Button. We need help. Hit the Emergency Code Button now." She hits the Emergency Code button, and we hear the overhead operator announce—*Code Team to Labor and Delivery. Code Team to Labor and Delivery.*

Chapter 22

Operating Room

As the hysteria continues around me, I instruct the paramedics to take Mrs. Johnson to the operating room. Paula stands in shock. Head Nurse Simmons grabs the out-of-control stretcher.

All eyes turn to me. I have to speak, "Push the stretcher into the operating room. Resident Saunders and Head Nurse Simmons, follow me. The rest of you take care of the injured boy."

We quickly follow the stretcher with Mrs. Johnson to the Operating Room. I yell down the hall, "I need one of the students to bring the ultrasound machine."

Dr. Green, the anesthesiologist, bends down to examine Micky. "The boy has shallow breathing and a faint pulse. Better get him down to the pediatric emergency room right away. Someone get the oxygen." Dr. Green then hurries to the operating room.

Nurse Pickens pulls a stretcher from the recovery room. Micky is gently lifted and placed on the stretcher. The Code Team arrives and transfers Micky to the pediatric emergency room.

I walk out of the operating room and yell down the hall, "Regina, call Dr. Carter in the ER, and let him know what happened here in Labor and Delivery."

◆◆◆◆◆◆◆◆◆◆◆◆◆◆◆◆◆◆◆◆◆◆◆◆◆◆◆

The team with the stretcher is in the operating room. I stop at the scrub sink and grab a surgical mask. I then hold it over my face and enter the surgical room. The first person I see is Surgical Scrub Technician Greg Jennings. I'm happy to see Greg. I have worked with him here in the past. He's very efficient, and he knows the instruments and procedures better than any of the doctors in training. He also has a great sense of humor. "Good to see you, Dr. Jones. I heard that you were coming back to the General."

I walk over to Greg. "News travels fast. I didn't even know I was coming back."

"Dr. Jones, things have not changed. Every time we meet, it's in the OR over some baby mama drama."

He's right, the first time I met Greg it was in the OR with a patient who had a liver rupture—talk about some scary baby mama drama. I can still remember the patient's face. Her last words on the table were, "Save my baby." We saved the baby but lost the mother. That was a really sad case. Losing mothers is never easy. Some things in life are really hard. Pregnant patients dying is one of them.

I walk over to Resident Saunders who's performing an ultrasound scan on Mrs. Johnson. "Resident Saunders what do we have here?"

"The ultrasound shows a thirty-two week fetus with a large blood clot behind the placenta. The baby is breech. The patient also has some vaginal bleeding. So far the heart tones are okay."

I look at the medical student who is standing beside Resident Saunders. "What is your name?"

"My name is John Richardson, and I am a third-year medical student."

"Future Doctor Richardson, what are the normal heart tones for a fetus?"

"The normal heart beat for a fetus is 120–160 beats per minute."

"Very good."

I look at Resident Saunders, "What is the diagnosis for this patient, Dr. Saunders?"

"Thirty-two week fetus, breech presentation, with a placenta abruption."

I look at the ultrasound screen. "You are correct. It is a placenta abruption—time to scrub." We walk out of the room and start scrubbing. The scrub sink is just as I remembered, no hot water. I look at the large dial in between the two scrub sinks. The handle is turned all the way to the right, labeled hot.

I look at Resident Saunders, "No hot water?"

"No ma'am, No hot water."

"Some things never change," I think to myself.

Resident Saunders then says, "We have this new waterless scrub system." He points to the bottle dispenser on the wall. "The hospital purchased that stuff last year. All the older doctors don't believe it works well enough to use in the operating room. It's okay for minor procedures, but major cases, the docs just don't use it. They don't think it kills bacteria well enough for surgery, so we continue to scrub with freezing cold water."

I look at the dispenser on the wall.

Resident Saunders continues, "I know freezing cold water doesn't kill bacteria either, so we are stuck between a rock and a hard place. Since I'm a second-year resident, I just do what my Attending does. If my Attending scrubs with freezing cold water, then I scrub with freezing cold water. If my Attending uses that waterless alcohol stuff that stinks and burns my skin, then I use it."

I say to myself, "He has a point—little twisted, but true. When in Rome do as the Romans do." My hands start to turn blue from the freezing cold water, and I begin to lose sensation in my fingertips.

I ask, "Do we have any information about this patient?"

"No, Dr. Jones, the only information we have on this patient is that she is the victim of a motor vehicle accident. Someone gave her some Demerol downstairs; she's been pretty out of it."

Resident Saunders tries to divert the question from himself and looks at Medical Student Richardson, "What is placental abruption?"

Medical Student Richardson tries to speak, "What is a placental abruption?" "Yes, you heard me. What is a placental abruption?"

"Don't know."

"You don't know? How long have you been on this OB rotation?"

Medical Student Richardson squeaks out the words, "Two days. Yesterday I spent the entire day in the OB clinic. We didn't talk about placental abruption."

Sensing the tension in the atmosphere, I say to Resident Saunders, "Resident Saunders this is a teaching service, not a pimping service. The medical students are here to learn. It is your job to teach them."

Resident Saunders looks at Medical Student Richardson.

"Resident Saunders, I believe you know what a placental abruption is… don't you?"

Resident Saunders looks at me with surprise, "Yes, Ma'am, I do."

Resident Saunders then turns to Medical Student Richardson and begins to speak, "The placenta is the life force for the fetus."

I finish my scrub and walk into the operating room.

Resident Saunders continues, "The placenta carries the blood from the mother to the baby. Twenty percent of the mother's blood supply goes to the placenta every minute. When the placenta starts to come off the wall of the uterus, it is called a placental abruption."

Medical Student Richardson commented, "That sounds serious."

"It's a life-threatening event for the mother and baby. If the placenta completely comes off the uterus, the mother can die in ten minutes. The baby can die in less than that."

"How did you know that this patient had a placental abruption?"

"We saw the blood clot on the ultrasound. The blood clot was located between the wall of the uterus and the placenta. The baby lives in water called amniotic fluid. Amniotic fluid shows up as black on the ultrasound machine. We saw a large white ball between the placenta and the wall of the uterus. That was the blood clot."

"Yes, I saw the white ball on ultrasound."

"Also, when I examined the patient she was bleeding vaginally."

Head Nurse Simmons opens the operating room door. "Better get a move on; the heart tones are falling. Last check, the heart tones were in the 80s."

"That is a sign that we have fetal distress."

"Placental abruption sounds serious."

"It is, you moron. If you ask me a question again in front of my Attending, I'll make sure *you* don't live long enough to finish this rotation. Number one rule: Always make your resident look good in front of the boss. If I look good, then you look good… Got it?"

"Got it."

"Now let's go. And remember, if I look good then you look good. Translation: don't ask me any freaking questions in surgery. I don't even want to hear you breathe. Got it?"

"Got it."

♦♦♦♦♦♦♦♦♦♦♦♦♦♦♦♦♦♦♦♦♦♦♦♦♦♦♦

My hands are finally beginning to thaw out as I put on my gown and gloves. I can now feel my fingertips.

"Where is my team?"

The circulating nurse looks out the door. "Here they come," she says.

Resident Saunders enters the room with Medical Student Richardson.

As the Medical Student is assisted with his gown and gloves, I say to him, "I take it you know all about placental abruption now?"

"Yes ma'am, Resident Saunders gave me a nice long lecture."

"Good for you, Resident Saunders. Let's get started and get this baby out. Dr. Green, my team is ready."

Dr. Green said, "She's asleep. You can cut."

A live baby boy is handed to the waiting Neonatal Intensive Care team.

Dr. Green says, "I am losing her blood pressure. Dr. Jones, what's going on down there? Her pressure is falling."

Dr. Green begins to instruct the team on resuscitation.

"Dr. Green, she's starting to bleed in her abdomen and I can't find the source. Better transfuse before we lose the patient."

Dr. Green orders the nurse, "Get me some blood products. Get me a central line. Move people. I need blood and a line today, not yesterday."

"I can't see. I need suction. I need some more sponges to clean the field. I can't see. I need another pair of hands."

Silence engulfs the room. It is as if I said something that was taboo.

Head Nurse Simmons tries to whisper, "Dr. Jones, all the other doctors are on strike. You're the only one here on Labor and Delivery."

"I'm sure Dr. Von is here. Someone page Dr. Von. I need her help. Someone get her here stat. I can't see. I need more suction. Dr. Green, she's just pouring out blood in her belly. I still can't tell where the bleeding is coming from."

The nursing staff scrambles to open up another suction device.

"I need some more laparotomy sponges. Better open up four more sets."

Head Nurse Simmons calls the front desk, "Regina, find Dr. Von. Tell her that Dr. Jones needs her in the OR stat."

Dr. Green warns, "Dr. Jones, her pressure is falling. We're losing her."

The medical student squeezes the bag of IV fluids to help the fluids run into the patient faster.

Dr. Green shouts, "Someone call the main OR and get Dr. Weber. Where is my central line kit?"

Head Nurse Simmons calls the front desk, "Regina, call the main OR and tell them Dr. Green needs Dr. Weber stat. Any word from Dr. Von?"

Clerk Regina replies, "Tell Dr. Jones that Dr. Von just called. She's on her way. Dr. Von should be walking through the Labor and Delivery Room doors any minute."

Dr. Green then looks at me. "Dr. Jones, any luck finding the source of bleeding?"

"Dr. Green, it looks like it's coming from above. I need to extend this incision."

Scrub Tech Greg places the scalpel in a basin and hands it to me.

Scrub Tech Greg, "Here you go, Dr. Jones, a size 10 blade."

"Thanks."

I quickly extend the midline incision up to the patient's breast bone. As I extend the incision, the blood gets worse and I can't see a thing.

"I need some help. I can't see."

The team does the best they can. Suction, sponges, suction, sponges.

I am operating like a mad woman. All I can think about is finding the source of bleeding and saving this patient's life. Blood is everywhere. The side pockets on the drapes are so full of blood that they are overflowing. The step stool that I am standing on is covered with blood, and I begin to lose my balance. The blood Dr. Green is transfusing into the patient is the same blood that I am seeing pour out and collect in the drapes. This is not good. This is a surgical nightmare, a bloody surgical nightmare.

Head Nurse Simmons grabs a sheet from the warmer and places it on the floor. "Here, Dr. Jones. Stand on this." I raise one foot and then the other. I lose my balance. I almost slip and fall. I focus. All my attention is on the bleeder. I have to find the bleeder. If I don't, this woman will die. She will just bleed out.

Dr. Green says, "The patient is hypotensive. We're losing her."

I have to concentrate. If I don't find this bleeder, then it will all be over. This lady's heart will have nothing to pump.

"I see it. I see the bleeder. It's bad. It's really bad. The pumper is coming from the spleen. The source of bleeding is the spleen. This is not good." I look up at Dr. Green.

I announce, "It is the spleen."

Dr. Green, without hesitation, says, "We need more blood products. Someone get them, move now. This patient is dying."

> The spleen is an ovoid mass about the size of one's fist. It is positioned behind the stomach and to the left of the kidney.

> The spleen is a major organ in the immune system and functions to filter unwanted elements from the blood.
>
> The spleen is very vascular. It has a large reserve pool of red blood cells (oxygen carrying cells), white blood cells (infection-fighting cells), and phagocytes (that remove damaged cells).
>
> The most common cause of injury to the spleen is a motor vehicle accident.
>
> Rupture of the spleen is followed by massive hemorrhage. If the spleen is *not repaired* or removed *promptly*, the patient can *die*.[6,12]

"Get me the Trauma Team and initiate the massive transfusion protocol. I need more blood. It is the patient's spleen. Someone page Trauma Team stat overhead."

Head Nurse Simmons calls the front desk. "Regina, we need the Trauma Team. Get them down here fast," she announces.

Dr. Green yells, "Where's my blood? Someone get me my blood."

Head Nurse Simmons, still on the phone, says, "Regina, Dr. Green needs the blood."

Clerk Regina reports, "The blood is on the way. Calling the Trauma Team now."

Nurse Pickens turns to Clerk Regina. "Sounds like they have a mess back there. Whatever it is, it doesn't sound good."

"You're right. Whatever is going on back there doesn't sound good. I have already called Dr. Von, the Blood Bank, and now the Trauma Team. Sounds like a zoo back there."

"With the strike today and all the docs gone, this is not good."

"You're telling me. Dr. Jones and Dr. Von are the only OBs in the hospital today? I don't know what we'll do if we have another emergency and they're still tied up."

"Regina, let's not think about it. You better call the paging operator and get the Trauma Team down here right away."

Clerk Regina calls the operator. "We have an emergency. Dr. Jones, the Attending, needs the Trauma Team on Labor and Delivery," she informs her.

The overhead paging operator activates all the trauma pagers and announces on the overhead pager.

> *Emergency*
> *Trauma Team to Labor and Delivery*
> *Emergency*
> *Trauma Team to Labor and Delivery*

Dr. Von walks through the doors of Labor and Delivery and asks, "Where is Dr. Jones?"

Clerk Regina replies, "Dr. Von, Dr. Jones needs you in Operating Room 1."

Dr. Von grabs a face mask, cap, and foot covers. She puts on a blue robe and walks into the operating room. She looks around. The room looks like a war zone. Blood and sponges are everywhere.

"Dr. Jones, what do you have here?"

"Dr. Von, it's the spleen. I'm applying direct pressure trying to slow down the bleeding until the Trauma Team arrives. It's not working too well. I have an approximate blood loss of three liters."

Medical Student Richardson informs us, "Total blood volume in an adult is five to six liters. This patient has lost half of her total blood volume."

Resident Saunders gives Medical Student Richardson a *shut-up look*.

Dr. Green looks at Dr. Von. "The patient is very hypotensive. She has lost a lot of blood. We have given her every blood product we have at this hospital, and we are still behind. I'm having problems maintaining her pressure. Dr. Von, the only thing that's going to save this patient's life is the removal of her spleen."

Dr. Von looks at Head Nurse Simmons. "Any word on the status of the Trauma Team?"

Head Nurse Simmons picks up the phone and calls the front desk. "Regina, any word on the Trauma Team?"

"The Trauma Team is in route. The team should be arriving through the Labor and Delivery doors any minute."

"Regina says the Trauma Team is on the way."

"They better get here fast. This lady is going down hill. If they don't hurry, she'll end up in the morgue with her spleen."

Dr. Green asks, "Any word on Dr. Weber?"

Head Nurse Simmons picks up the phone to call Clerk Regina.

Chapter 23

Trauma Surgeons

The Trauma Surgeons arrive in Labor and Delivery and are directed to the operating room. Dr. Gage enters the room and immediately starts barking out commands. "What is the problem? I have patients in my office, and I have a very busy schedule. Why was I summoned to Labor and Delivery like a common criminal? Paged overhead so the whole hospital knows I have been summoned? What is the freaking emergency?"

I look up at Dr. Gage. "This patient is dying on the table."

"And how is that my problem? Aren't you a surgeon?"

"It is the spleen. Dr. Gage, you are the trauma surgeon. The spleen is your domain."

"How do you know that it is the spleen?"

I ignore the hostility and continue to give the report. "The patient is a victim of a motor vehicle accident. She presented to us with a placenta abruption. Once I removed the baby, the uterus contracted, and the patient began to hemorrhage. The bleeding was coming from the abdomen, so I extended the incision. That is when I noticed it was the spleen."

"Why are you just now calling me for help?"

"The pregnant uterus was keeping the bleeding under control. The patient started to bleed after we removed the baby."

Dr. Green turns to Dr. Gage and intervenes, "This patient is unstable, and we need some help. You can finish this 'Surgeons Walk on Water' conversation later."

Dr. Gage mutters, "Why is she not in the main operating room with proper equipment and adequate staffing? This place looks like a prehistoric dinosaur. No staff... no surgical equipment..." He looks at the suture material, "Cat Gut Chromic. This stuff looks like rope. No respectable surgeon would be caught dead using this stuff. I cannot believe you guys are still killing cats and using their guts to make suture material. Cat Gut Chromic, how archaic! Move the patient downstairs to a more suitable operating room. I will go now and assemble my team."

Dr. Green looks up from the patient, "Dr. Gage, this patient cannot be moved. She is dying on the table. We need you to do something like operate, take out her spleen, and save her life. Get in here and do something."

"You expect me to operate in this room with no equipment? It is like operating in the jungle. Move her downstairs to a more functional and standard of care operating room. I would not operate on my pet fish in this place."

"The patient is dying; we can argue about what operating room another time. We can continue this conversation and any other grievances you have with the Hospital Sanctions Committee later."

Dr. Gage looks at Head Nurse Simmons. He relents, "Call the main operating room and have my special instruments brought up. I also need my Surgical Scrub Nurse Bantana up here. Get me some real suture material, none of that Cat Gut stuff. Still killing cats. I should call the Humane Society."

Dr. Gage storms out of the room to scrub and soon returns. "Nurse, I need an extra large gown, and I wear two pairs of size ten gloves. I want a pair of Latex-free gloves on the bottom and the plain gloves on top," he demands.

"Any other barking orders?"

Scrub Tech Greg answers, "Ruff, Ruff."

Dr. Gage says, "This place is full of comedians. Everybody has jokes."

Surgical Scrub Nurse Bantana enters the room with the surgical instruments. Head Nurse Simmons walks over to Surgical Scrub Nurse Bantana. "I will take that for you," she says, "What size gloves do you wear?"

"I wear two size six gloves."

"Do you want any latex-free gloves?"

"No, two pair of plains are fine for me." Surgical Scrub Nurse Bantana then walks out to the scrub sink.

Dr. Gage looks at Head Nurse Simmons. "What is the status of the consent?"

Head Nurse Simmons starts to fumble through the chart.

"You do have a signed consent form, Dr. Jones, don't you?"

"Dr. Gage, what part of unstable did you not understand? The patient was in a motor vehicle accident. Last time I checked, they were not using consents in the jungle."

Dr. Gage then turns his attention to the patient. "You can move your hands now, Dr. Jones," he says, "You and your team can get the hell out of the way, or you can stay and learn something about real surgery." Dr. Gage continues with a hint of sarcasm, "Your domain is between the belly button and the knees. I know you don't know anything about real surgery in the abdomen. I am amazed you could identify the spleen."

I remove my hands and step back out of the field. I want to say something so bad, but I think about the patient. No matter how cantankerous Dr. Gage may be, he is still the one to remove this patient's spleen. Right now, saving this lady's life is all that counts.

After I remove my hands, Mrs. Johnson begins to hemorrhage. Dr. Gage explores the surgical site and then announces, "This spleen is damaged beyond repair. It has to go."

"Finally, we agree on something." I bite my lip. I want to say, "I told you so."

Dr. Green announces, "I am losing her blood pressure. Dr. Gage, do something."

Dr. Gage replies, "I am working in suboptimal conditions in a hostile environment with incompetent staff. What do you expect me to do? My last name is not Houdini."

The student nurse in the corner whispers to her colleague, "Can't he just tie off something?"

Dr. Gage looks up: "Quiet! This is not the time to entertain nonessential personnel. Get those damn students out of here. Remove them now. I mean now."

Nurse Kelly rushes all the students out of the room. The Neonatology Transport Team also leaves with the baby. Dr. Gage begins to remove the spleen.

Chapter 24

No Prenatal Care

During the removal of Mrs. Johnson's spleen, another patient arrives on Labor and Delivery in a wheelchair.

Clerk Regina calls for the Charge Nurse over the speaker.

Nurse Spectra tells her, "Charge Nurse Simmons is still in the Operating Room."

Nurse Spectra looks at the patient in the wheelchair. The patient begins to faint, so the nurse instructs the transporter to wheel the patient into Labor Room 1.

"Regina, we need the doctor stat."

Medical Student Tom helps Nurse Spectra lift the patient out of the wheelchair and onto the bed. As the patient is lifted out of the chair, a pool of blood begins to drip onto the floor.

Nurse Spectra says, "This patient needs to go to the Operating Room. Help me take her to Operating Room 2."

Intern Doctor Lowery comes into the room. "What do we have here?"

Nurse Spectra answers, "The patient just arrived. She's bleeding. We need to take her to Operating Room 2."

Intern Lowery turns to the medical student saying, "Tom, you grab the ultrasound machine and follow me."

Nurse Spectra says, "The ultrasound machine is already in the back. It's in Operating Room 1."

The patient is quickly taken to the back. Medical Student Tom walks into Operating Room 1 and grabs the ultrasound machine. While there, Tom says, "Dr. Jones, Doctor Lowery needs you in Operating Room 2."

Everyone looks at Medical Student Tom.

"Operating Room 2? What is going on next door?"

"You don't know? Doctor Lowery just told me to get you and the ultrasound machine."

Dr. Gage is still very busy removing the spleen. I look up at Dr. Green and Dr. Weber. "I will be next door."

Dr. Weber (anesthesiologist) says, "I better come with you. Sounds like you are going to need anesthesia."

Dr. Weber and I walk into Operating Room 2.

Intern Lowery turns on the ultrasound machine and begins to scan the patient. "Dr. Lowery, what is the story?"

"The patient came in and collapsed."

We both look at the ultrasound machine. The screen shows a full-term baby with a small amount of fluid. A large blood clot is seen between the uterus and the placenta. The heart tones are in the 80s. They are low.

Intern Lowery says, "…Looks like a placental abruption with fetal distress."

Medical Student Tom with a puzzled look asks, "What is a placental abruption?"

Intern Lowery answers, "A placental abruption is when the placenta becomes detached from the wall of the uterus. Since the placenta supplies the fetus with blood, if the placenta completely detaches from the wall of the uterus the fetus and mother can die within a matter of minutes. A placental abruption is a life-threatening emergency, and they usually come in threes."

"What do you mean by threes?"

"The patient next door had a placenta abruption. This is the second patient for the day. We will probably see one more within the next twenty-four hours."

Dr. Weber announces, "Dr. Jones, you can cut in two minutes."

Head Nurse Simmons walks into the room saying, "You cannot operate now. I don't have the staffing. I would have to pull one of my nurses from the floor to work as the circulator, and I need another nurse to scrub. I cannot tie up two Operating Rooms. What if a patient comes in with another trauma? You have to wait. I don't have the staffing."

Dr. Weber looks at Head Nurse Simmons and yells, "What do you think this is? We have an emergency right in front of our eyes. We don't have to wait for another one to come crashing through the doors."

"Nurse Simmons we have to operate. I know you can make it happen. We are going to scrub and save this baby's life. We have no options."

Dr. Weber snaps, "I bet you won't tell that to the judge. I see the headlines now—Patient died at the General because Nurse Simmons said *no staffing*."

Head Nurse Simmons calls Student Nurse Tonya into the room. This is Tonya's second day on Labor and Delivery and her first day in the operating room.

"Tonya, I need you to circulate so I can scrub with the doctors."

Student Nurse Tonya is then instructed to pull the gowns and gloves from the cabinets for the doctors.

Resident Doctor Tremor walks into the room and begins to help open the instruments. Dr. Weber has difficulty placing the tube in the patient's airway. The alarm for the oxygen attached to the patient's finger begins to beep.

Beeeep!

The patient's oxygen content begins to fall, and Dr. Weber immediately attempts to ventilate the patient using bag ventilation. I look up at Dr. Weber and see the panic on his face.

With a mother in trouble and the baby's life in jeopardy, I say, "Scalpel."

The patient begins to move violently in an attempt to free herself from the table.

Intern Lowery says, "She's moving. The patient is trying to get off the table."

"Hold her down. I can't cut on a moving target."

Medical Student Tom tries to hold the patient down. He is unsuccessful. The patient again tries to free herself and begins to move violently on the table. Tom grabs one leg but is unable to reach the other. The free leg strikes the instrument tray. The instruments go tumbling to the floor.

Cling! Clang! Cling! Clang!

Everyone looks on in disbelief as the instruments continue to tumble onto the floor.

"I need a scalpel right away; this baby is in trouble. I need to cut. This baby will die if I don't get it out," I shout.

Head Nurse Simmons tells Tonya, "I need you to pull a scalpel from the cabinet. The scalpels are in the top drawer."

Student Nurse Tonya locates the scalpel and hands it to Head Nurse Simmons.

Chapter 25

Operating Room 1

Dr. Gage announces, "My team is finished. The patient's incision is ready to be closed by the OB team."

Dr. Green reminds him, "The OB team is busy next door."

"You would think they have more than one doctor up here competent enough to perform surgery."

Nurse Francis says, "The doctors are on strike. Dr. Gage, isn't your wife, Dr. Trent-Gage, one of the doctors on strike?"

Dr. Gage gives Nurse Francis a condescending look. "The location and professional status of my wife are none of your damn business," he says between gritted teeth.

Dr. Gage looks at the incision and says, "This incision looks like it was made by a butcher. The incision is the only part of the surgery the patient sees. I will not be blamed for this hatchet job. Let the butcher that made it, close it. Go get the butcher."

Dr. Gage rips off his gown and gloves. He throws them on the floor, tramples on them, and storms out the room.

Nurse Francis mutters, "Good riddance. I've seen some pretty incisions, but the patient died, and I've seen some ugly incisions, and the patient lived. I'll take an ugly incision with life any day. I'm sure Mrs. Johnson won't be too upset when she wakes up from anesthesia and finds out that she and her baby are both alive."

Scrub Tech Greg agrees, "Got that right. Give me life with an ugly incision any day."

Greg looks down at the incision and says, "I know this was an emergency and Dr. Jones was working under pressure, but this is a jacked-up incision. Dr. Gage was right. Looks like it was made by a butcher. A not-so-happy one at that."

Nurse Francis says, "Greg leave the patient alone. Do you need me to open up anything for the closure."

Scrub Tech Greg says, "Better wait until Dr. Jones gets back. I don't remember what she uses to close."

All the student nurses walk back into the room.

Dr. Green sends Student Nurse Kelly to Operating Room 2 instructing her, "Find out how much longer the team will be in surgery."

Student Nurse Kelly walks into Operating Room 2 saying, "Dr. Jones, Dr. Green wants to know how much longer you will be? They need you next door."

"Tell Dr. Green I am waiting on an X-ray. I will be right there."

Student Nurse Kelly walks into Operating Room 1 and informs everyone, "They're waiting for X-ray next door. Dr. Jones said that she's on her way."

Student Nurse Lisa asks, "Why are they waiting for an X-ray next door?"

Nurse Francis explains, "When you have emergency surgery, the instruments are not counted before the surgery. An X-ray is ordered to make sure nothing is left inside the patient. The patient can only be closed after the X-ray report is read as negative. So, they're waiting next door to close the patient."

I open the door to Operating Room 1.

Dr. Green explains, "Dr. Gage stormed out of the room, and the patient still needs her incision closed."

"I will do a quick scrub and be right there. Nurse Francis, pull out another gown for me."

Scrub Tech Greg asks me, "Dr. Jones what do you want for closure? I have one medium staple gun on the table."

"That should be enough. I will be right there."

As I walk to the scrub sink, I think to myself, "Another freezing cold scrub." After a quick scrub, I walk back into Operating Room 1.

Relieved, Scrub Tech Greg says, "Dr. Jones, we're glad you're back. Dr. Gage kept ranting and raving. He was throwing instruments and blaming everyone else for his little-man shortcomings. It was crazy… Just pure madness. Gage was out of control."

I explore the surgical site and then close the incision. I look up at Dr. Green and say, "The surgery is complete. Time to get out of here."

"Sounds good to me. Dr. Jones, better send the patient down to the Surgical Intensive Care Unit. Total blood loss is six liters."

"Six liters? When I left the room the count was three liters."

Surgical Scrub Tech Greg pipes up, "I told you it was crazy. Dr. Gage kept ranting and raving that the patient's spleen was enlarged. He kept shouting, 'extra blood volume, huge vessels, no normal anatomy.' He was off the chain, and it was a blood bath. You see this room."

Dr. Green says, "I have totally replaced this patient's entire blood volume. She has no circulating blood of her own in her body."

Scrub Tech Greg adds, "This lady completely wiped out the entire blood bank. If another patient comes in, we'll have to get blood from another hospital."

Dr. Green tells me, "Better call SICU for a bed."

"Good idea. I will go and talk to the family. I will be back to escort her down to the unit. What floor is the surgical unit on?"

"The surgical unit is on the fourth floor. The emergency elevators open directly into the unit."

Nurse Spectra enters the room and tells me, "X-ray cleared."

I return to the room and close the incision. The patient is taken to the recovery room in a stable condition.

Chapter 26

Mrs. Crane Returns

Mrs. Crane returns to Labor and Delivery because she is having severe contractions. All eyes are on her as she is wheeled to the front desk. Mrs. Crane relives the events of earlier and says, "I don't want to be here. I don't want to be back here where Micky was hurt."

Head Nurse Simmons tells the aide, "Escort Mrs. Crane to Labor Room 4. Regina, page Dr. Jones and the resident."

I walk up to the nursing station with Intern Doctor Lowery.

Clerk Regina says, "Dr. Jones, guess who's back?"

"Who is back?"

"It's Mrs. Crane, and she looks pretty bad."

"Regina, how is her son?"

"Don't know. She just came in and was wheeled into Labor Room 4."

I walk into the room with Intern Doctor Lowery and Medical Student Tom. We stare at the fetal monitor and say, "Mrs. Crane, looks like you are having contractions every two minutes."

"I don't want to be here. I want to be with my son."

Intern Lowery puts on a pair of gloves and examines Mrs. Crane. "The patient's cervix is dilated 2–3 centimeters, and the head is low in the birth canal," he says.

"We need to stop her labor."

"I am only six months pregnant. It is too early for the baby to come. When I left, I was told I was having Braxton Hicks contractions. They said all I needed was some fluids. I just need some IV fluids," Mrs. Crane informs us.

"Mrs. Crane you are now in true labor, and we need to stop your contractions."

Attorney Crane enters the room. "Dr. Jones, how are my wife and son doing?" he asks.

"Your wife is going into true labor, and the baby is premature. I will be starting medication, magnesium sulfate, to stop the contractions. If I cannot stop the labor, your baby has less than a ten percent chance of survival."

"Doctor, do what you can to save my baby."

"Mr. Crane, we will do our best for your wife and your baby."

I walk out of the room. I feel a sharp chest pain. I stop and grab the wall. I take a few shallow breaths, and the pain goes away. I look up and see the neurosurgeons walk through the labor room doors.

Chapter 27

Neurosurgeons

Dr. Thomas and his team walk onto Labor and Delivery. Clerk Regina asks him, "Can I help you?"

"I am looking for the parents of Michael Crane."

"The patient is in Labor Room 4."

I walk out of Labor Room 4 and towards the nursing station.

"Dr. Thomas, Dr. Jones is the Attending Physician for Mrs. Crane. Here she comes now," the clerk informs Dr. Thomas.

"Hello Dr. Jones," he says, "I need to talk to the parents of Michael Crane. The patient has a massive bleed and needs to have emergency surgery."

I escort the team into Labor Room 4. As we enter the room, we find Attorney Crane standing over his wife and wiping her forehead with a cold cloth. He looks up as we walk through the door.

"Attorney Crane, this is Dr. Thomas, the head of the Neurosurgery Division here at Mercy General Hospital. Dr. Thomas is taking care of your son."

"A neurosurgeon? Why is a neurosurgeon taking care of my son?"

"Dr. Thomas has some important information to discuss with you and your wife."

Attorney Crane gently shakes his wife and wakes her up, "Honey, the doctors are here to talk about Micky."

Mrs. Crane looks at me and then looks at Dr. Thomas.

"Hello, my name is Dr. Thomas, and I am a neurosurgeon. I was called by Dr. Carter in the emergency room to evaluate your son, Michael Crane. Can you tell me what happened to him?"

Attorney Crane explains, "He was hit by a stretcher here on Labor and Delivery."

Mrs. Crane begins to cry. She again relives the accident. "How is my son, doctor?" she asks through her tears.

"As you know, your son is in a coma. He is now starting to have seizures, and we are having a difficult time controlling them. The CT scan of your son's head reveals bleeding and swelling in the brain."

"What are you telling us doctor? Is Micky going to die?"

"He is critical. I need to operate to save your son's life. I know this is a very difficult time."

Attorney Crane says, "My wife asked you a question. Is Micky going to die?"

"We plan to do our best to save him. I wish I had more to offer, but I will not know until we operate. I have contacted Dr. Farnsworth from the Vanderbilt to assist me. He is the best neurosurgeon in the country."

Attorney Crane says, "Dr. Peter Farnsworth is our neighbor and is a good friend of the family. I really appreciate you calling him."

"I would like to go over the surgical consent."

"I am an attorney, a medical malpractice attorney, and I won a 250-million-dollar judgment from this hospital. I want to know everything that you plan to do to my son. I mean everything. I want to know 250 million dollars' worth of information. Got it?"

Dr. Thomas takes a deep breath. "Mr. Crane, the procedure is called an exploratory craniotomy with the evacuation of a hematoma and damaged brain tissue."

"Explain the procedure in a manner my wife can understand."

Medical Student Tom pulls out his notepad.

"At surgery, the hair over the damaged area is shaved. An incision is made into the scalp. The bone is taken out in a single flap and will be replaced after surgery. The blood clot and damaged brain tissue will be removed. If the brain is very swollen, I may decide not to replace the skull bone. Following the surgery, I will place an intracranial pressure catheter that will give us a constant reading of the pressure inside of the skull."

Dr. Peter Farnsworth walks into the room. He immediately walks over to Attorney Crane.

Attorney Crane tells him, "Peter, I am so glad you are here."

"I am so sorry that it has to be under these circumstances. Dr. Thomas called me to assist him. I came from the Vanderbilt as soon as I got the message."

Dr. Thomas adds, "Thanks for coming Peter. Attorney Crane, do you have any other questions?"

"When can I see my son? I want to see him before the surgery."

"He is getting prepared for surgery now. I will have someone take you to the holding area."

Mrs. Crane begs, "I need to see my son. Take me to see Micky."

Head Nurse Simmons gently says, "Mrs. Crane, I need you to calm down."

Mrs. Crane then pulls the IV out of her arm and tries to sit up. Head Nurse Simmons opens the gauze and holds pressure on Mrs. Crane's arm to stop the bleeding.

Attorney Crane firmly tells her, "Honey, you have to stay here and take care of this baby. I will go and be with Micky. It is going to be ok."

Attorney Crane then signs his name on the consent form. He looks at Dr. Thomas. "I trust you with my son's life. Do what needs to be done."

"We will."

Dr. Farnsworth adds, "We both will."

Head Nurse Simmons replaces the IV and gives Mrs. Crane some sedation. Mrs. Crane quickly falls asleep.

Chapter 28

Operating Room

Attorney Crane is standing by the stretcher in the holding area. Dr. Thomas tells him it is time for his son, Michael Crane, to be wheeled into the Operating Room. Attorney Crane bends over and kisses his son, Micky, on the forehead. He looks up at Dr. Thomas and Dr. Farnsworth. "Please take care of my son. Please take care of Micky!" he pleads.

Dr. Thomas assures him, "I will come and find you as soon as the surgery is over."

Micky is then taken into the Operating Room and placed on the surgical table.

Nurse Carter asks, "Is this the boy who was injured upstairs?"

Nurse Riley says, "Yes, he's the one who was hit by a stretcher. I was told his mother is on Labor and Delivery, having her baby."

"How horrible for the family."

While the doctors are scrubbing, Dr. Farnsworth tells Dr. Thomas, "I have not been over here since my training days."

"Yes, it has been a long time. Hard to believe we were residents here together over twenty-five years ago."

"This is unbelievable. The Cranes have been neighbors for a long time. I remember when this boy was born."

"It is a tragedy. I am glad you are here."

"This family is special to me. I am glad you called. Time to get started."

The surgery begins. A portion of the skull is removed, and the brain is explored.

"I found the bleeder. It is coming from an aneurysm. The boy has a bleeding aneurysm."

"Are you able to control the bleeding with a clip?"

"I think I can get it." Dr. Thomas places a clip but it doesn't work; the bleeding continues. "Load the clip again. I think I can get it," Dr. Thomas instructs.

Dr. Weber (anesthesiologist) cuts in, "The patient is becoming unstable. His pressure is falling, and I am losing his pulse."

"Try to place the clip from your side."

Dr. Farnsworth fires the clip… No good. The patient continues to bleed.

Dr. Weber again says, "His pressure is falling. I am losing him."

Dr. Farnsworth says, "We have to pack the bleeding for now and come back later."

"Whatever you do, do it quick. He is going downhill fast—*we've lost sinus rhythm!*"

Dr. Thomas instructs the circulating nurse, "Start chest compressions. Where is the crash cart?"

Dr. Thomas looks at the rhythm strip. He grabs the paddles of the defibrillator. "Charge. Stand Clear!"

Dr. Thomas places the paddles from the defibrillator on Micky's chest.

Dr. Weber says, "No change on the rhythm strip."

"Charge. Stand Clear!"

Dr. Thomas again shocks the patient.

Dr. Weber states, "No change on the rhythm strip."

"Charge. Stand Clear!"

Dr. Thomas again shocks the patient.

Dr. Weber pushes epinephrine and then atropine through the IV line.

A coldness enters the room. The room is filled with a mixture of sadness and disbelief. No one speaks, and no one moves. Dr. Thomas looks down at the patient.

Dr. Thomas says, "The patient is too unstable to continue the operation."

Dr. Farnsworth concurs, "I agree, better get him to the unit. I only hope that the compression from the packing continues to stop the bleeding. We just did not know about that aneurysm. If only we knew the bleeding was coming from an aneurysm we could have approached it differently. Why didn't it show up on the CT scan?"

The surgery is stopped, and the patient is transferred to the Surgical Intensive Care Unit. Dr. Farnsworth puts a hand on the shoulder of Dr. Thomas. "We did our best. The damage was too extensive. The boy is just too unstable. We just did not know about the aneurysm."

Dr. Thomas says, "There was no history of headaches, seizures, or black-out spells. The family said the boy was perfectly healthy. It was not seen on plain CT because the large blood clot was in the way. The aneurysm would have been seen on the MRI."

"Why didn't you order a MRI?"

"The MRI machine is down for repairs."

"That is not good. MRI is the standard of care."

Dr. Thomas says, "I know."

Dr. Farnsworth tells him, "Think on the bright side. The boy was born with this condition. He had no symptoms and no previous head imagining studies. We had no way of knowing he had an aneurysm."

Dr. Thomas replies, "Think on the bad side. His father is a medical malpractice lawyer."

"A very successful malpractice attorney who won a 250-million judgment from the General last year."

"Time to go and find the Crane Family."

"I don't know how they will take this news. The boy may never come out of the coma."

"I know, the boy may never wake up."

Chapter 29

Labor and Delivery

Dr. Thomas and Dr. Farnsworth walk onto Labor and Delivery. Dr. Thomas tells Clerk Regina, "I need to speak to Dr. Jones."

"Dr. Thomas, is the Crane boy alright?"

"I need to speak to Dr. Jones."

"You can wait in Labor Room 2, right over there. I'll page Dr. Jones for you."

Dr. Thomas and Dr. Farnsworth walk into Labor Room 2.

"Dr. Jones to Nursing Station. Dr. Jones to Nursing Station."

I walk out of Labor Room 4 and up to the nursing station.

"Yes, did someone page me?"

"Dr. Jones, the neurosurgeons want to talk to you. They are waiting for you in Labor Room 2. They seem really uptight. I just know that something bad has happened. You'd better go quickly."

I walk into Labor Room 2 and can feel the tension in the room. "Dr. Thomas, Dr. Farnsworth, how is the Crane boy?" I ask.

Dr. Farnsworth tells me, "Not good. It is not good."

Dr. Thomas adds, "The patient's brain injury was more extensive than we realized. When we got in, we found out that the boy had an aneurysm that must have ruptured as a result of the accident with the stretcher. The aneurysm ruptured, and all hell broke loose. It was a bloody mess."

Dr. Farnsworth added, "We just could not control the bleeding. We clipped the aneurysm, but he is still bleeding. He coded on the table, so we had to end the surgery."

I stare in disbelief. "Where is the boy now?"

Dr. Farnsworth says, "He is in the Surgical Intensive Care Unit."

Dr. Thomas adds, "That aneurysm could have ruptured anytime and anywhere: at home, at his school, at the playground. Of all places, it had to rupture from a stretcher at the General... Talk about bad luck."

Dr. Farnsworth says, "Luck for the patient—can you imagine what would have happened if he had not been in the hospital? He might have died on the way here. I would say lucky for the patient, but unlucky for the hospital."

I tell them, "The Crane family is in Labor Room 4. I believe Attorney Crane is there with his wife. I will come with you to talk with them." I escort Dr. Thomas and Dr. Farnsworth into the Labor Room 4.

Mrs. Crane looks up and immediately senses something is wrong. With tears in her eyes, she says, "How is my son? How is Micky? Is the surgery over? Where is my son, Micky?"

Dr. Thomas starts, "I am sorry to have to tell you this ..."

Mrs. Crane begins to scream. "Micky! No, not Micky!" She screams so loud that the entire Labor and Delivery Ward can hear her cry.

Dr. Thomas continues, "The brain injury was more extensive than we thought. Your son had an aneurysm."

Dr. Farnsworth adds, "He was born with an aneurysm. It is a congenital anomaly."

Attorney Crane asks, "What is an aneurysm?"

Dr. Thomas answers, "An aneurysm is a bulge or dilation that occurs in a weak area of a blood vessel."

Mrs. Crane exclaimed, "How can this be? My son was never sick?"

"When your son was struck, the weak area in the blood vessel ruptured and caused massive internal bleeding. We were unable to control the bleeding in the operating room..."

Attorney Crane interrupts, "What are you saying?"

"Your son's heart stopped, and we could not continue with the surgery. It was too risky to continue. Micky's heart was too weak."

Attorney Crane asks, "Where is my son? I want to see my son."

Attorney Crane then walks over to Dr. Thomas, "Leave us! Get out! I said leave us!" he shouts.

All medical staff leave the room. The cries and ear-piercing screams of Attorney and Mrs. Crane can be heard down the hall.

Back at the desk, Clerk Regina tells me, "Dr. Jones, you got a call from a Dr. Timmons in the emergency room. He just said you need to page him right away. I knew you were in counsel with the Crane family, so I did not disturb you. Dr. Timmons said it was really important."

"Thanks, Regina. Would you call him for me?"

Clerk Regina calls the Emergency Room. "Hello, this is Labor and Delivery. Dr. Timmons wants to speak to Dr. Jones."

ER Clerk Evilyna answers, "Dr. Timmons is with a patient."

"I am calling for Dr. Jones."

Labor and Delivery

"Yeah, yeah… Dr. Timmons said for her to come down here and pick up her old lady."

"Her mother! Did you say her mother?"

"Da….Uh….Do you have hearing problems? I said tell the doctor to come and pick up her old lady. It is crazy busy down here and we need the room. If she doesn't get down here soon, we will park the old hag in the lobby."

"Are you sure you want to speak to Dr. Jones on Labor and Delivery."

"You heard me. Tell the doc to come and get this old woman!" says ER Clerk Evilyna slamming down the phone.

Clerk Regina hangs up the phone and then looks at Head Nurse Simmons, "I don't think Dr. Jones knows."

"Knows what?"

"That was the ER on the phone. Dr. Jones' mother is there as a patient."

"Really?"

"Yes, and Evilyna said her mother is ready for discharge."

"Here comes Dr. Jones. You better tell her."

"I can't. You tell her. I just can't do it. I can't lie to her with a straight face."

"And you think I can?"

"Yes, you can. Here she comes. Tell her."

Head Nurse Simmons tells me, "Dr. Jones, Dr. Timmons wants to see you in the ER right away."

"Did Dr. Timmons tell you what the problem is?"

"No, he just said for you to come right away."

"Okay, I am on my way. Regina, page the Chief Resident, and have the Resident meet me in the ER."

"I don't think they want to see the Chief Resident."

"What did you say Regina?"

"She did not say anything, Dr. Jones."

I walk to the ER.

Head Nurse Simmons whispers, "Regina, that was close."

"I told you; you can lie with a straight face. You did good."

"Regina, your big mouth is going to get us all in trouble one day."

"Sorry. I didn't mean to say anything. It just slipped out. I feel terrible."

"Imagine how Dr. Jones is going to feel when she finds out about her mother."

Chapter 30

Emergency Room

I walk into the emergency room.

Dr. Timmons asks, "Are you Dr. Jones from OB/GYN?"

"Yes, I am."

"Is your mother Mrs. Elouise Jones?"

My heart drops. I am paralyzed. I am in shock. Did he just say my mother's name, Elouise Jones? I hold my breath as I wait for the next sentence. I am now an emotional wreck, and my heart begins to race.

Dr. Timmons reads the panic on my face. He inquires again, "Are you related to Mrs. Elouise Jones?"

"Yes, I am. She is my mother."

"Dr. Jones, your mother was brought in earlier today. She was in a motor vehicle accident. She is waiting for you in the triage holding area."

I walk into the room. My mother looks at me with such sadness. "I am sorry to bother you. I did not mean to hurt anyone," she says.

"Mom, what are you talking about? It is okay. Mom, it is okay."

I walk over to my mother and lay my hand on her shoulder.

"I did not see the light. It all happened so fast."

Dr. Timmons says, "Your mother is free to go. I want her to check in with her doctor in a couple of days."

"Thanks, Dr. Timmons."

My pager goes off. I look down. It is Labor and Delivery.

"Mom, I will be right back. I have to answer this page."

As I walk out the door, another sharp chest pain hits me. I stand still and hold my breath.

A nurse asks me, "Doctor, are you okay?"

"Yes, thank you. I need to use the phone and call Labor and Delivery."

"You can use the house phone over there."

Chapter 31

Cliffhanger

As I stand next to the hospital phone, I find it hard to believe the events of the day. My mind starts to spin out of control. I just came to the General to speak to Dr. Von about a part-time job, and I walk into all this.

Baby Mamma Drama

Hospital Strike:	*Administration vs. OB Staff over Family Center Care Policy.*
Mrs. Johnson:	*Motor vehicle accident patient who almost died on the table. Her life was saved when Dr. Gage removed her spleen.*
Michael Crane:	*Hit by the stretcher carrying Mrs. Johnson. He had emergency surgery and is now in a coma, fighting for his life.*
Mrs. Crane:	*Preterm labor. If she delivers, her baby has less than a ten percent chance of survival.*
Mother:	*Motor vehicle accident, treated in the emergency room. Thank God she is all right and ready for discharge.*
Me:	*Have completed Two emergency surgeries and am now dealing with recurrent episodes of chest pain.*

My pager goes off. I look down at the number. It is Labor and Delivery. A deep pit fills the bottom of my stomach. The pager goes off again. This time it is Labor and Delivery calling with the 911 code.

> 911 Labor and Delivery
> 911 Labor and Delivery

This is not good. It must be the Crane baby. All this drama is enough to give a normal person with no heart problems chest pain. So guess what is happening to me?

To be continued…

Appendix

1. Medical Definitions
2. Medical Specialist
3. Medications
4. Medical Abbreviations
5. Medical Organizations
6. References

Medical Definitions[13]

Amniotic Fluid: Liquid that surrounds the growing fetus. Produced from the amnion.

Anemia: A reduction in the number of red blood cells in the blood.

Aneurysm: A localized blood-filled dilation that occurs in a weak area of a blood vessel.

Angioplasty: Mechanical widening of a narrowed or obstructed blood vessel.

Ballottement: A technique that is used to examine a floating object. A tap with the fingers causes the fetus to move away and then to return as it floats back to the original position.

Blood Components

Red Blood Cell (Erythrocyte): Cell containing hemoglobin. Principal function is to transport oxygen. Dysfunction will lead to anemia.

White Blood Cell (Leukocyte): Cell of the immune system that helps the body fight against infectious disease or foreign materials. Dysfunction will lead to infection.

Platelets (Thrombocyte): Cell fragments that form blood clots. Dysfunction will lead to bleeding.

Phagocyte: A cell that ingests and destroys foreign material. Dysfunction can lead to infection.

Fibrinogen: A protein used in blood clot formation. Dysfunction can lead to bleeding.

Blood Pressure: The force exerted on the walls of your blood vessels as blood flows through them. Optimal blood pressure with respect to cardiovascular risk is 120/80. A healthy individual can tolerate blood pressure between 90/50 and 135/90.

Brachial Plexus: A network of nerves that originate near the neck and transmit signals from the spine to the shoulder, arm, and hand.

Breech: The position of the baby in the womb when it is not head down.

Caffeine: A drug that has a stimulant action on the central nervous system. It is used to help people stay awake. This drug has diuretic properties that can lead to an increase in urination.

Cancer: A disorder of uncontrolled cell division leading to a tumor. Can affect any area of the body. May grow by direct contact with other cells (invasion) or by distant sites (metastasis).

Cervix: Lowest portion of the womb that dilates for childbirth.

Cesarean Section (Delivery): Delivery of fetus through the abdomen.

Clinical Pelvimetry: Measurement of the birth canal.

Coma: A state in which the person can not be aroused.

Computerized Tomography (CT): A radiology technique that involves recording slices of the body with an X-ray scanner.

Congenital Anomaly: A birth defect that occurs in the womb.

Contusion: A bruise, caused by blunt trauma, in which capillaries are damaged and blood is allowed to move into adjacent tissues.

Cord Prolapse: Umbilical cord delivering through the cervix before the fetus.

Craniotomy: Surgical operation in which part of the skull is removed.

Death: Permanent cessation of vital functions.

Brain Death: Irreversible damage to the centers of the brainstem that control breathing and other vital reflexes. Once the patient has been declared brain dead, organs may be legally removed for transplantation surgery before the heart has stopped. Requires two independent medical opinions.

Defibrillator: An electromagnetic device that applies an electric shock to restore the normal rhythm of the heart.

Diabetes Mellitus: A disorder characterized by high blood sugar (hyperglycemia). Complications can lead to blindness, renal failure, eye damage, heart disease, nerve damage, gangrene, or coma.

Echocardiogram: Ultrasound of the heart.

External Cephalic Version: A process by which the fetus is gently guided into the head-down position via abdominal massage and pressure.

Fetal Demise: Death of a fetus greater than 20 weeks gestational age or of a weight in excess of 500 grams.

Fundus: The part of the uterus above the uterine tubes. The part farthest from the birth cannel. The top of the uterus.

Group Beta Streptococcus: A Gram-positive, nonmotile, bacteria that occurs in chains. The bacteria have the ability to destroy red blood cells (hemolysis). Infection in a newborn can lead to pneumonia or meningitis.

Head Entrapment: Fetal head caught in birth canal. Can lead to difficulty with the delivery and possible fetal damage.

Hematoma: A mass of clotted blood that forms in the tissue.

Hemorrhage: Medical term for bleeding. The human body generates two liters of blood per week.

Hydration: Replacement of fluid.

Hypertension: High blood pressure. Blood pressure >140/90. Complications can lead to damage to the eye or kidney, and can cause a heart attack or stroke.

Hypotension: Low blood pressure. A small drop in blood pressure, even as little as 20 mm/Hg can lead to lightheadedness and dizziness. Complications can lead to fainting and seizures.

Intravenous (IV): Entering by way of a vein.

Intubation: Placement of a tube into the body.

Labor and Delivery: Facility where pregnant women are evaluated and give birth.

Last Menstrual Period: The menstrual period dated from the first day of the last normal menstrual period.

Magnetic Resonance Imagining (MRI): A radiology technique that involves recording slices of the body with a magnetic scanner.

Menstruation: A cyclic event under hormonal control that leads to the physiologic discharge of blood and mucosal tissues from the non-pregnant uterus. Normal cycles occur every four weeks.

Neonatal Intensive Care Unit: Critical care area for the evaluation and treatment of infants first born and within the first four weeks of life.

Nuchal Arm: Fetal arm is trapped around the back of the neck. Releasing one or both arms by force may lead to a fracture of the humerus.

Obstetrical Triage Area: Facility for the initial evaluation of pregnant women.

Ophthalmoscope: Instrument used to examine the eye.

Otoscope: Instrument used to examine the ear.

Postpartum: The period following childbirth that extends to approximately six weeks.

Preterm Delivery: Delivery of the fetus before 38 completed weeks of pregnancy.

Preterm Labor: Uterine contractions that lead to cervical change before 38 completed weeks of the mother's last menstrual period (LMP).

Seizure: An abnormal electrical discharge in the brain leading to sensory disturbances, convulsions, or loss of consciousness.

Spleen: Organ that functions to filter unwanted elements from the blood.

Stethoscope: An instrument used to listen to sounds within the body.

Tocolysis: Medication used to suppress labor.

Ultrasound Machine: A machine that uses ultrasounds (sound waves > 20,000 Hz inaudible to the human ear) to produce images of things within the body.

Umbilical Cord: A cord arising from the navel that connects the fetus with the placenta for the exchange of nutrients and waste products.

Uterus: Female womb. Major reproductive organ in the body.

Term Delivery: Delivery of a fetus that is greater than 38 completed weeks from the mother's last menstrual period (LMP).

Medical Specialists[13]

Doctors
Medical Student: Medical school trainee.
Intern: First year medical graduate.
Resident: Physician who is receiving specialty training in a hospital.
Attending Physician: Physician who has completed specialty training.

Anesthesiologist: A medical specialist who provides relief of pain (anesthesia).

Cardiologist: A medical specialist who provides care and treatment of the heart.

Emergency Medical Services: Medical personnel who provide care and treatment of the acutely ill or injured person.

Gynecologist: A medical specialist who provides care and treatment to females.

Intensive Care Unit: Area in hospital where critically ill patients are treated.

Neonatal Intensive Care Unit: Critical care area where newborns are treated.

Surgical Intensive Care Unit: Critical care area for patients who have undergone surgery.

Maternal-Fetal Medicine: A medical specialist who provides care to high-risk pregnant patients.

Medical Oncologist: A medical specialist who provides care to cancer patients.

Midwife: A nurse practitioner who specializes in normal child birth.

Neonatologist: A medical specialist who provides treatment and care to newborn babies.

Obstetrician: A medical specialist who provides care to pregnant patients.

Pediatrician: A medical specialist who provides care to children.

Paramedic: A specially trained medical technician who provides a wide range of emergency services before or during transportation to the hospital.

Surgeon: A medical specialist who performs operations.

General Surgeon: An individual who manages all surgical problems. Work is not restricted to a specific area.

Neurosurgeon: An individual who manages surgical problems involving the brain and spinal cord.

Trauma Surgeon: An individual who manages emergency surgical problems.

Medications[13]

Ambien: Used for sleeping disorders (insomnia) because it has hypnotic properties.

Atropine: Used in the treatment of low heart rate. Blocks the parasympathetic nervous system and speeds up the heart.

Chlorpheniramine: An antihistamine used for cold symptoms and sinus congestion.

Codeine: A narcotic used for pain control that has anti-cough (antitussive) properties.

Demerol: A narcotic used for pain control.

Epinephrine: A fight or flight hormone that is released from the adrenal glands whenever danger threatens. Used as a drug to shunt blood away from the peripheral area and back to the heart.

Hydrocodone: A narcotic used for pain control.

Morphine: A narcotic used for pain control.

Naloxone: A narcotic antagonist. Used to reverse the effects of narcotic drugs.

Narcotic: A drug derived from opium. It is used to decrease pain, induce sleep, and alter mood or behavior.

Penicillin: An antibiotic that is used to kill susceptible bacteria.

Pitocin: A form of oxytocin that is used to contract the uterus.

Robitussin: A narcotic derivative that is used to suppress coughs.

Tussionex: A narcotic derivative that is used to suppress coughs.

Tylenol: An analgesic and antipyretic. A pain control medication that lowers a fever.

Medical Abbreviations[13]

CPR   Cardiopulmonary resuscitation

CT   Computerized tomography

GYN   Gynecology

IV   Intravenous

LMP   Last menstrual period

MRI   Magnetic resonance imagining

SICU   Surgical intensive care unit

NICU   Neonatal intensive care unit

OB   Obstetrics

Helpful Medical Organizations

American Academy of Pediatrics www.aap.org

American Cancer Society www.cancer.org

American College of OB/GYN www.acog.org

American College of Surgeons www.facs.org

American Diabetes Association www.diabetes.org

American Heart Association www.americanheart.org

Helpful Website

Wikipedia—Free encyclopedia www.wikipedia.org

References

1. Wikipedia. www.wikipedia.org.

2. *The Merck Manual of Medical Information.* Home Ed. 2nd ed. Simon & Schuster, 2003. 100-117.

3. *Physician's Desk Reference*: PDR 2007. 61st ed. Montvale, NJ: Thomson PDR, 2007. 3227.

4. Cunningham, Gilstrap, Levono et al., Williams Obstetrics, 22nd ed., McGraw-Hill, 2005.

5. *Student's Life Application Study Bible.* Carol Stream, Ill.: Tyndale House Publishers, 2004. 1017.

6. Moore, Keith L., and Arthur F. Dalley. *Clinically Oriented Anatomy*. 5th Ed., International ed. Philadelphia, Pa.; London: Wolters Kluwer Health/Lippincott Williams & Wilkins, 2006. 281-286.

7. Gabbe, Niebyl, Simpson., Pocket Companion to Accompany Obstetrics: Normal and Problem Pregnancies. 4th ed. New York: Churchill Livingstone, 2002.

8. *Rapid Response to Everyday Emergencies: A Nurse's Guide.* Lippincott, Williams, and Wilkins Company, 2006, 1-8.

9. American Heart Association *Advanced Cardiac Life Support Textbook*, 1994, 1-10.

10. American College of Obstetricians and Gynecologist: *Breast Cancer Screening*: Practice Bulletin Number 42, April 2003, pages 299-300.

11. Beckmann, Charles R. B. *Obstetrics and Gynecology*. 3rd ed. Philadelphia, PA: Lippincott Williams & Wilkins, 1998.

12. Cotran, Ramzi S., and Vinay Kumar. *Robbins Pathologic Basis of Disease*. 3rd ed. Philadelphia: Saunders, 1989.

13. Bantam Medical Dictionary, Bantam edition ed. 1981.

CPSIA information can be obtained
at www.ICGtesting.com
Printed in the USA
BVHW060204231220
596053BV00002B/5